Clinical Judgment

Robert L. Schalock, PhD

Hastings College

Ruth Luckasson, JD

University of New Mexico

D1520604

AAMR

American Association on Mental Retardation

Published by
American Association on Mental Retardation
444 North Capitol Street, NW
Suite 846
Washington, DC 20001-1512

The points of view expressed herein are those of the authors and do not necessarily represent the official policy or opinion of the American Association on Mental Retardation. Publication does not imply endorsement by the editor, the association, or its individual members.

Printed in the United States of America

Library of Congress Cataloging-in-Publication Data

Clinical judgment / Robert L. Schalock, Ruth Luckasson.
    p. cm.
Includes bibliographical references and index.
ISBN 0-940898-89-6
1. Clinical medicine--Decision making. 2. Mental retardation--Diagnosis. 3. Medical logic. 4. Medicine--Decision making. I. Schalock, Robert L. II. Luckasson, Ruth.

 R723.C557 2005
 616.85'88--dc22
                          2005045333

Contents

Tables

Figures

Preface

We have written this book for at least three reasons.

First, our combined experiences in the field of mental retardation over the past 30 years have shown that, when making decisions and demonstrating best practices, clinicians use more than research-based knowledge, professional standards, and professional ethics. Some refer to this ancillary "thing" as intuition, some as one's better judgment, some as blind faith, and some as professional license. We consider the "thing" to be clinical judgment—a special type of judgment rooted in a high level of clinical expertise and experience and based on extensive data. These characteristics of clinical judgment not only separate it from intuition, blind faith, or professional license, but also augment the three other competencies involved in best practices: research-based knowledge, professional standards, and professional ethics.

Second, we have written this book because the field needs it. Increasingly, clinicians working with individuals with mental retardation are expected to make decisions requiring a level of competence regarding clinical judgment strategies, guidelines, and actions that extends beyond their formal training. Service recipients and their individualized support needs are different today than even a decade ago. The community-based and self-advocacy movements present clinicians with new challenges and require decisions regarding inclusion, equity, and empowerment. Similarly, the service delivery system continues to change, with its focus on personalized supports, brokered services and supports, and increased demands for accountability. Additionally, the "system" is both more complex and less "tight." Sometimes clinicians are asked to make decisions based on incomplete information, often because of linguistic and/or cultural diversity and restricted opportunities for thorough assessment, interviews, and observations. What do we do when confronted with less than optimal assessment information, complex medical and/or behavioral conditions, legal restrictions, and/or cultural diversity? To overcome these challenges successfully, the field needs to become more familiar with the clinical judgment strategies, actions, and guidelines described in this book.

Third, we have written the book for the future. We believe that the changes we are experiencing are but the tip of the iceberg. Our clientele will continue to change; the challenges and opportunities presented by their desire for lives of personal satisfaction and well-being will increase our need to become more familiar with them and their environments. Similarly the service delivery system will challenge us to implement more fully the supports paradigm, including the evaluation of valued outcomes related to the provision of individualized supports. And finally the provision of best practices will necessitate clinical judgment strategies in which a clinician should be competent—strategies related to: conducting thorough social histories; aligning data collection to the critical questions asked by multiple stakeholders; applying broad-based assessment strategies; implementing intervention strategies based on descriptive, functional, ecological, and outcome analyses; planning, implementing, and evaluating individualized supports; and reflecting cultural competence and linguistic diversity.

We hope and anticipate that by reading this book professionals will become better clinicians. Although we understand and appreciate the critical roles that research-based knowledge, professional standards, and professional ethics play in our work with individuals with mental retardation, our experiences confirm the need to add a fourth component to best practices—clinical judgment. Clinical judgment is not an excuse for poor practices or a way to solve political problems. Rather, as you are about to see, it is a special type of judgment reflected in specific strategies, actions, and guidelines to ensure competence. Its overall purpose is to improve best practices in the field of mental retardation.

Robert L. Schalock
Ruth Luckasson
April 2005

PART 1
Context and Framework

Best practices in the field of mental retardation are based on research-based knowledge combined with professional ethics, professional standards, and clinical judgment. The overall purpose of clinical judgment is to ensure best practices. The use of clinical judgment in a particular case enhances the precision, accuracy, and integrity of the clinician's decisions. As introduced here in part 1, clinical judgment is rooted in a high level of clinical expertise and experience. It emerges directly from extensive data and is based on (a) the clinician's explicit training, (b) direct experience with individual clients, and (c) specific knowledge of a particular person and the person's environment.

Clinical judgment is different from either ethical or professional judgment. Ethical judgment is generally concerned with judgments of value and obligation focusing on justice (treating all people equitably), beneficence (doing good), and autonomy (respecting the authority of every person to control actions that primarily affect him- or herself). Professional judgment is a process that follows specific professional guidelines by which a member of that profession collects, organizes, and weighs information. In distinction, clinical judgment relies on six strategies related to assessment, intervention, and cultural and linguistic competence. Furthermore, it is characterized by its being systematic (i.e., organized, sequential, and logical), formal (i.e., explicit and reasoned), and transparent (i.e., apparent and communicated clearly).

Here in part 1, we provide an overview of clinical judgment, including the strategies and operational actions that help ensure a competent clinical judgment, appropriate guidelines to use in reference to each of six clinical judgment strategies, and the

1

importance of understanding clearly the focus of a question set before you, the skills that are needed to answer the question, and the question's anticipated product. In addition, we compare clinical judgment to professional ethics and standards, propose that clinical judgment is based on researched-based knowledge, and discuss core disability concepts that are the basis of current services and supports to people with mental retardation. Once the context and framework of clinical judgment are well understood, the reader will be in a good position to continue with part 2, an in-depth analysis of each of the six clinical judgment strategies. Part 3 gives further insight into the clinical judgment process and its incorporation into best practices.

CHAPTER 1

An Overview of Clinical Judgment in Mental Retardation

Context

As clinicians in the field of mental retardation, we all experience situations that challenge us personally and professionally. Sometimes the situations involve evaluations we are asked to perform; others involve intervention strategies we are asked to develop; and still others involve professional or expert opinions requested of us. In each case we rely on research-based knowledge, professional practices and standards, and professional codes of ethics. But we also rely on something else—clinical judgment, even though we might not have been able to articulate clearly what it is.

Think back on situations where you had to rely on "clinical judgment." We authors think of times when parental rights were an issue; when it was necessary to determine the impact of severe burns on the quality of life of a person diagnosed as "profoundly retarded"; when a positive behavior support program needed to be developed for an individual whose positive behaviors, according to many peers and staff, were nonexistent; when a thorough social history was required in a case involving the criminal justice system; when a broad assessment strategy was used to establish eligibility for special education services; when cultural and linguistic diversity was critical in diagnosis and eligibility determination.

It is safe to say that our professional training did not prepare us well enough to make all the complex and challenging decisions set before us. Frequently we have needed more than research-based

3

knowledge, professional standards, and professional codes of ethics; indeed, we needed the fourth component of best practices: clinical judgment. We needed that special type of judgment rooted in a high level of clinical expertise and experience; the type of judgment that emerges directly from extensive data. This book is about this fourth competency involved in best practices—clinical judgment—and what it is, and what it is not.

The need for a book on clinical judgment in the field of mental retardation is critical today because of trends impacting the field, principally: (a) the power struggle and shifting alliances between self-advocates and professionals; (b) the competing models of disability, such as ecological, trait, and functional; (c) the conflicting values among stakeholders in the inclusion and empowerment movements; (d) questions about the modern application of traditional scientific approaches; (e) conflicting models of resource allocation; and (f) challenges to the future of traditional professionals. These trends, either singularly or in the aggregate, explain why now there is the need to explicate clinical judgment.

Although the need for this book is apparent in today's complex world of questions that are hard to answer, its development has been slow. Its time has come, for a number of reasons, including:

- the inclusion of people with mental retardation into the mainstream of life, which raises significant and frequently hard-to-answer questions about rights and responsibilities;
- the subjective and personal-well-being revolutions with their emphasis on a life of quality and opportunities for personally satisfying lives;
- the supports paradigm with its emphasis on determining the profile and intensity of needed supports and interfacing services with the natural environment;
- the multicultural nature of clientele that frequently presents challenges regarding the need to understand and accept different attitudes, beliefs, and behaviors;
- the emergence of transdisciplinary teams with the corresponding deemphasis on "disciplinary autonomy" (Menand, 2001);

- the increased involvement of people with mental retardation in the legal system and the challenges inherent in assessment and adjudication;
- the emergence of the reform movement with its emphasis on accountability and data-based decision making.

Clinical judgment is not just a phrase to throw around, as some do. How often, for example, have you heard someone (even an expert) say, "My opinion is based on clinical judgment"? As you read this book, you will find that, as one of the four competencies composing best practices, clinical judgment involves strategies, operational actions, and guidelines. You will also find that clinical judgment is an essential component of good decision making and best practices. Finally you may find that it is something you have been using but did not name.

The remainder of this chapter defines clinical judgment and places it in the context of best practices within the field of mental retardation. In that regard, we feel that clinicians who can best use clinical judgment are those with: training and expertise in mental retardation, extensive relevant assessment data, ongoing experience with the particular person involved, ongoing experiences and observation of individuals with mental retardation and their specific environments, and ongoing experience with individuals with mental retardation and their families.

Purpose, Definition, and Contraindications

Purpose of Clinical Judgment

The overall purpose of clinical judgment is to ensure best practices. The use of clinical judgment in a particular case enhances the precision, accuracy, and integrity of the clinician's decisions in that case.

Definition of Clinical Judgment

Clinical judgment is a special type of judgment rooted in a high level of clinical expertise and experience; it emerges directly from extensive data. It is based on the clinician's explicit training, direct experience with those with whom the clinician is working, and specific knowledge of the person and the person's environment. Competent clinical judgment is based on the specific strategies, operational actions, and guidelines discussed in this chapter. Clinical judgment is characterized by its being: (a) systematic (i.e., organized, sequential, and logical), (b) formal (i.e., explicit and reasoned), and (c) transparent (i.e., apparent and communicated clearly).

Contraindications of Clinical Judgment

Clinical judgment should not be thought of as a justification for abbreviated evaluations, a vehicle for stereotypes or prejudices, a substitute for insufficiently explored questions, an excuse for incomplete or missing data, or a way to solve political problems.

Clinical Judgment as a Part of Best Practices

Clinical Judgment Compared to Professional Ethics and Standards

Clinical judgment is different from either ethical or professional judgment based on one's professional ethics and standards. Ethical judgment is generally concerned with judgments of value and obligation focusing on justice (treating all people equitably), beneficence (doing good), and autonomy (respecting the authority of every person to control actions that primarily affect him- or herself). Professional judgment is a process that follows specific professional guidelines by which a member of that profession collects, organizes, and weighs information. In distinction, clinical judgment is a special type of judgment rooted in a high level of clinical expertise and experience and is based on the use of specific strategies, actions, and guidelines. It emerges directly from extensive data and is based on training, experiences, and specific knowledge of the person and his or her environment.

Our reading of a number of organizational documents regarding professional ethics suggests strongly that most ethical guidelines can be integrated into the following five ethical principles: (a) exhibits competence, (b) exhibits professional and scientific responsibility, (c) shows respect for peoples' rights and dignity, (d) exhibits concern for others' welfare, and (e) contributes to community and society. Although each profession may define these principles slightly differently, collectively these five principles encompass well the purpose of a profession having a set of ethical principles, which is to describe: (a) a system of moral behavior and (b) the rules of conduct recognized in respect to a particular class of human actions or a particular group.

Thus, a primary use of a professional code of ethics is to provide a framework for the internal monitoring of a profession as a whole. Another primary use is that it also provides the partial basis for: evaluating practices and personnel preparation, accrediting or certifying education and habilitation programs, reviewing professional behavior, and enforcing rules of conduct.

Generally each profession also publishes professional standards associated with each of its professional ethical principles. These professional standards provide the basis for evaluating practices and personnel preparation and are used for accreditation or quality control; as a measure against which to compare individual performance; and/or as criteria to review professional behavior and enforce rules of conduct. Thus, for example, in reference to the ethic of competence, associated professional standards relate to: (a) maintaining knowledge of current scientific and professional information regarding services rendered and (b) participating in the objective and systematic evaluation of themselves, colleagues, and services for the purpose of continuous improvement of professional performance. In Table 1.1 we show the relationship among clinical judgment strategies and the professional ethics and professional standards gleaned from our review of professional organizations' documents. As clearly shown, each clinical judgment strategy is embedded in professional ethics and standards. As noted earlier, however, clinical judgment is not the same as professional ethics and standards.

Table 1.1

Relationship Among Clinical Judgment Strategies and Professional Ethics and Standards

---

Strategy 1: Conducting a thorough social history

- Ethical principles: competence, professional and scientific responsibility, respect for people's rights and dignity, concern for others' welfare
- Professional standards: boundaries of competence, objective judgment, client and professional relationships, records, conflict of interest, individual differences, informed consent, human rights, misuse of information, power relationships, attitude barriers

Strategy 2: Aligning data and its collection to the critical questions at hand

- Ethical principles: competence, professional and scientific responsibility, respect for people's rights and dignity, concern of others' welfare, contributes to community and society
- Professional standards: current information, objective judgment, records, individual differences, disclosures, misuse of information, scientific investigations, personal and social well-being

Strategy 3: Applying broad-based assessment strategies

- Ethical principles: competence, professional responsibility, respect for people's rights and dignity, concern for others' welfare
- Professional standards: current information, boundaries of competence, services offered, referrals, objective judgment, diagnostic and test procedures, public statements, personal responsibility, records, conflict of interest, individual differences, revealed information, disclosures, informed consent, misuse of information

Strategy 4: Implementing intervention best practices

- Ethical principles: competence, professional and scientific

---

responsibility, respect for people's rights and dignity, concern for others' welfare

- Professional standards: current information, boundaries of competence, services offered, objective judgment, client relationships, records, individual differences, revealed information, disclosure, informed consent, human rights, misuse of information, scientific investigations

Strategy 5: Planning, implementing, and evaluating individualized supports

- Ethical principles: competence, professional and scientific responsibility, respect for people's rights and dignity, concern for others' welfare, contributes to community and society
- Professional standards: current information, service delivery and practice, client relationships, personal responsibility, records, individual differences, self-determination, human rights, advocacy, personal and social well-being

Strategy 6: Reflecting cultural competence and linguistic diversity

- Professional ethics: competency, professional and scientific responsibility, respect for people's rights and dignity, concern for others' welfare, contributes to community and society
- Professional standards: boundaries of competence, objective judgment, client relationships, diagnostic tests and procedures, personal responsibility, conflict of interest, individual differences, human rights, power relationships, attitude barriers, service improvement

Note: Based on an analysis and synthesis of the following published codes of ethics: American Geriatrics Society (2001), American Medical Association (2001), American Nurses Association (2002), American Psychological Association (1992; 2002), American Speech-Language-Hearing Association (2003), Benjamin & Curtis (1992), Howe & Miramontes (1992), National Association of Social Workers (1996), National Board of Certified Counselors (1997), National Career Development Association (2003), National Education Association (1975), Reinders (2002), and Vehmas (2004).

Relation of Clinical Judgment to Best Practices

The relationship among research-based knowledge, professional ethics, professional standards, and clinical judgment is shown in Figure 1.1. Clinical judgment plays a variable role in best practices. The amount of emphasis on clinical judgment will vary depending on the amount of information, type of information, complexity of the issue, and the qualifications, experience, and expertise of the clinician. Thus some clinical judgments are more structured than others. For example, an emergency situation where an experienced nurse triages on the basis of experience and expertise is quite different from a situation where a clinician makes a clinical decision regarding the legal competency of a person based on incomplete information. Situational factors that result in uncertainty, imprecision, ambiguity, and complexity require an increased application of clinical judgment. However, in some situations, even clinical judgment cannot legitimate an assessment.

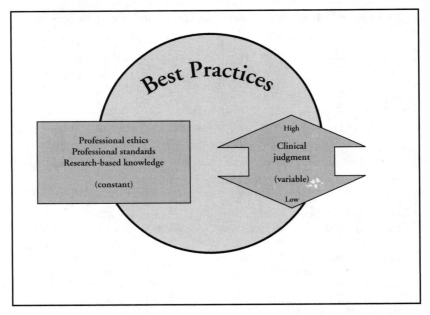

Figure 1.1. Role of clinical judgment in best practices.

In summary, clinical judgment is an essential component of best practices and enhances the accuracy of decision making in complex situations involving diagnosis, classification, supports provision, and practice-based evidence. Clinical judgment not only enhances best practices, but it also provides a professional framework for decision making. This framework is explained more fully in the following sections.

Clinical Judgment Based on Research-Based Knowledge

Best practices in the field of mental retardation are based on professional ethics, professional standards, clinical judgment, and research-based knowledge. In reference to research-based knowledge, over the past decade we have seen significant changes in how we pursue knowledge about the condition of mental retardation. Our research methods have expanded to include: (a) the use of both quantitative and qualitative approaches to gather information, (b) a focus on the social ecology of behavior, (c) an understanding of the genetic-neurochemcial mechanisms involved in the condition, (d) the emphasis on early intervention programs and their effects, (e) the use of multivariate and causal model research designs to determine significant predictors of desired outcomes, and (f) the analysis of public policies.

Collapsing across these techniques, six research trends have emerged that have—and will continue to have—a significant impact on the field of mental retardation and the increased need to use clinical judgment:

1. an ongoing investigation of brain-behavior relationships (Warren, 2002);

2. a further elaboration of the role of genetic and neuro-biochemcial mechanisms in the expression of mental retardation (Henderson, 2004);

3. a multidimensional approach to etiology that stresses a multifactorial and intergenerational model of mental retardation etiology and prevention (Luckasson et al., 2002);

4. the emerging disability paradigm, with four characteristics focusing on functional behavior, personal well-being, individualized supports, and personal competence (Schalock, 2004);

5. an evaluation of the impact of public policies and judicial decisions on the lives of individuals with mental retardation (Herr, O'Sullivan, & Hogan, 2002); and

6. the evaluation of the core concepts of disability policy summarized in Table 1.2 (Turnbull, Wilcox, Stowe, & Umbarger, 2001).

These six research trends and the research-based knowledge underlying them will undoubtedly increase our understanding of the condition of mental retardation and its amelioration; they will also influence how best practices are defined and evaluated. Each of these trends will raise ethical issues about prevention, intervention, and human rights. Thus they will affect professional practices, standards, and guidelines regarding how one collects, organizes, and weighs information. Of direct relevance to readers of this book, they will also increase the use of clinical judgment as clinicians will face the need to: conduct thorough social histories; align data and its collection to the critical questions asked; apply broad-based assessment strategies; implement intervention best practices; plan, implement, and evaluate individualized supports; and reflect cultural competence and linguistic diversity. With increased knowledge, questions will become more complex and will require not just more information, but also the alignment of multiple data sources to the questions asked and the decisions required.

As a part of research-based knowledge, clinicians also need to be aware of disability core concepts. Disability policy in the United States is embedded in a number of core concepts that are reflected in federal statutes that generally have corresponding state statutes. One or more of the eight core concepts summarized in Table 1.2 will affect professionals making decisions that demonstrate best practices: antidiscrimination, individualized and appropriate services, diagnosis, capacity-based services, empowerment or participatory decision making, service coordination and collaboration, integration, and productivity and contribution (Turnbull et al., 2001).

Table 1.2
Core Concepts of Disability Policy

Antidiscrimination: Refers to equal treatment, equal opportunity, and accommodation. Principal federal statutory sources include Rehabilitation Act (1973); Americans With Disabilities Act (ADA; 1990); and Individuals With Disabilities Education Act (IDEA; 2004).

Individualized and appropriate services: Refers to services that are specially tailored to meet the needs and choices of individuals with disabilities and their families. Principal federal statutory sources include IDEA; ADA; Rehabilitation Act (§ 504); Children's and Communities Mental Health Systems and Improvement Act (1994); Omnibus Budget Reconciliation Act (1987); and Developmental Disabilities Assistance and Bill of Rights Act (2000).

Diagnosis: Includes processes and criteria by which a person with a disability becomes eligible for benefits or services. Principal federal statutory sources include Supplemental Security Income for the Aged, Blind, and Disabled (Title XVI of the Social Security Act; 1972); Rehabilitation Act; Developmental Disabilities Assistance and Bill of Rights Act; Children's and Communities Mental Health Systems and Improvement Act; Home Care for Certain Disabled Children (Katie Beckett) Waivers (1994); and IDEA.

Capacity-based services: Involves the evaluation of the unique strengths and needs of the person. Evaluation includes choices, resources, priorities, and concerns along with the identification of services necessary to enhance family and individual capacity. Principal federal statutory sources include IDEA; Rehabilitation Act; Children's and Communities Mental Health Systems and Improvement Act; and Adoption Assistance and Child Welfare Act (1980).

Continues on page 14

Empowerment or participatory decision making: Involves the constitutional principles of autonomy, choice, consent, privacy, and liberty as grounded in the 1st and 14th Amendments. Principal federal statutory sources include IDEA; Developmental Disabilities Assistance and Bill of Rights Act; and Rehabilitation Act.

Service coordination and collaboration: Includes activities that assist individuals or their families to access and benefit from services and supports from more than one agency (interagency) or within a single provider system (intraagency). Principal federal statutory sources include IDEA; Assistive Technology Act (1998); Children's and Communities Mental Health Systems and Improvement Act, and Child Health Act (2000).

Integration: Includes integration and inclusion into least restrictive environments with appropriate supports. Principal federal statutory sources include IDEA; Title XIX (Home and Community Based Services [HCBS] Waiver) of the Social Security Act (1971); Developmental Disabilities Assistance and Bill of Rights Act; ADA; and Rehabilitation Act.

Productivity and contribution: Refers to engagement in meaningful human activity such as, for example, income-producing work and unpaid work that contributes to household or community. Principal federal statutory sources include Developmental Disabilities Assistance and Bill of Rights Act; Rehabilitation Act; ADA; Workforce Investment Partnership Act (1998); IDEA; Goals 2000: Educate America Act (1994); Improving America's Schools Act (1994); Ticket to Work and Work Incentives Improvement Act (1999); and Title XIX (HCBS Waivers) of the Social Security Act.

Adapted from Turnbull, Wilcox, Stowe, and Umbarger (2001).

A number of core concepts discussed by Turnbull et al. are not included here, because they relate more to the ethical principles and professional standards summarized in Table 1.1. These concepts include protection from harm, liberty, privacy and confidentiality, family integrity and unity, cultural responsiveness, accountability, professional and systems capacity, and prevention and amelioration.

Knowledge of these eight core concepts of disability policy will directly affect clinicians and the clinical judgments and decisions they make. Clinicians must realize that people should be free from discrimination, are entitled to individualized and appropriate service and supports, are empowered to participate in the mainstream of life, and make decisions about factors that impact their personal well-being. As for diagnosis and classification, it is equally important for clinicians in their judgment and decision-making roles to ensure that evaluations focus on: the person's limitations and needs; the person's unique strengths; the incorporation of choices, resources, practices; and identification of services and supports that are necessary to enhance individual and family capacity.

Situations That Typically Require Clinical Judgment

Put yourself in the following situation: The call came, as they frequently do, out of nowhere. The district court judge on the line introduced himself and stated very judiciously, "I need your professional opinion. I have this case involving parental rights. The person central to the case is a single parent, mentally retarded, and an African American. Can you help? I can see you tomorrow morning at ten. Would that be OK?" Yes, you'll be there.

Although clinical judgment is always required, a number of situations—such as that reflected in the judge's call—necessitate a heightened reliance on clinical judgment to enhance decision making and facilitate best practices. These situations typically occur when:

- **Formal assessment is less than optimal** (e.g., unreliable, invalid, incomplete, inappropriate) and cannot be improved but, even so, may be sufficient to provide a partial basis for making

15

clinical judgment.

- **Complex medical or behavioral conditions require multiple analyses** (e.g., descriptive, functional, ecological, outcome) that must be balanced in the application of clinical judgment.

- **Legal restrictions significantly impact opportunities to assess the person** consistent with the five assumptions of the definition of mental retardation. These five assumptions are

  1. Limitations in present functioning must be considered within the context of community environments typical of the individual's age peers and culture.

  2. Valid assessment considers cultural and linguistic diversity as well as differences in communication, sensory, motor, and behavioral factors.

  3. Within an individual, limitations often coexist with strengths.

  4. An important purpose of describing limitations is to develop a profile of needed supports.

  5. With appropriate supports over a sustained period, the life functioning of the person with mental retardation generally will improve. (Luckasson et al., 2002, p. 1)

  When such restrictions are operative, the application of clinical judgment can proceed if there is a substantially equivalent data base established through one or more of the strategies discussed in the next section.

- **Cultural diversity and/or linguistic factors impact or affect the information needed for decisions.** Consideration of those cultural and/or linguistic factors will require clinical judgment.

  Assisting the district court judge in reaching a decision regarding the person's parental rights required clinical judgment (as will be shown clearly in chap. 7). As one might guess, however, there was a story behind the story. Over the phone the judge did not explain the pressure he was receiving from the local social service agency, the individual's neighbors, and the family, which desired foster placement for the child. During the morning meeting, it was apparent that there was a paucity of assessment information, other than "she's retarded and has been in special education." It also became apparent that the immediate family wanted nothing to do with the child and "those welfare people." This example reflects commonly occurring situations that require the use of those strategies discussed next.

Competent Clinical Judgment: Six Strategies

The four situations listed in the previous section require the use of one or more of the six clinical judgment strategies summarized in Table 1.3. Although each strategy is the focus of one chapter in part 2, the following brief description of each will be helpful to the clinician who is facing one or more of these four situations.

Table 1.3 Competent Clinical Judgment: Six Strategies
1. Conducting a thorough social history
2. Aligning data and its collection to the critical question(s) at hand
3. Applying broad-based assessment strategies
4. Implementing intervention best practices
5. Planning, implementing, and evaluating individualized supports
6. Reflecting cultural competence and linguistic diversity

Conducting a Thorough Social History

A social history must do more than describe the significant events in a person's life. Rather, a thorough social history will address issues related the individual's past, present, and future. In addition, it will take a wholistic approach that focuses on both the individual's strengths and limitations. A thorough social history will help a clinician formulate hypotheses about present and future behaviors and life situations. Compiling a thorough social history is always an important part of a diagnosis, but it is especially critical when a retroactive diagnosis is sought or when the stakes are high. In the case of most children today, compiling the social history is relatively easy because of mandated school records and the presence of the family. In the case of adults who have not previously had a diagnosis, however, compiling the thorough social history will demand more time and resources. If the stakes are very high, as in many legal and guardianship cases, considerable care and attention will be necessary to exercise good clinical judgment.

Aligning Data and Its Collection to the Critical Question(s) at Hand
Clinicians, as others, often find themselves being "data rich and information poor." This situation suggests strongly that much information collected is of dubious value and frequently not aligned with either the question(s) needing to be answered or a clear conceptual framework. So how does one align data and its collection to the critical question(s) at hand?

The first step is to understand clearly the focus of the question you're being asked to answer. (We'll discuss this further in chap. 2, which explicates the first of six operational actions—clarify the question). Our experience suggests that three types of questions are most frequently asked of clinicians: those related to diagnosis, classification, or planning supports. Given this, the critical question(s) is aligned to data and data collection as follows:

• For diagnosis-related questions, essential data relate to intellectual and adaptive behavior functioning and age of onset.

• For classification-related questions, essential data relate to competency indicators, needed support indices, intelligence subdomains, adaptive behavior domain profiles, and etiology risk-factor analysis.

• For planning-supports-related questions, essential data relate to profiles of needed supports and their intensity and outcomes from the assessment of objective life conditions.

The second step in aligning data to the posited question(s) is verifying that the measures and data collection strategies used are in line with best practices, according to criteria such as: (a) the match between measures and purpose; (b) acceptable psychometric properties of the measures selected (especially in regard to reliability and validity); (c) the appropriateness for the person in regard to age and cultural group, primary language, means of communication, gender, and sensori-motor limitations; (d) examiner characteristics and potential bias; (e) selection of informants; (f) relevance of context and environments; and (g) physical, behavioral, and mental factors potentially impacting the assessment situation.

Applying Broad-Based Assessment Strategies

Because of the clinician's inability to evaluate the person on a standardized test, it is sometimes necessary to develop a working hypothesis or diagnosis. Thus an essential clinical judgment strategy is to apply broad-based assessment techniques when the person is either nonverbal or emotionally impaired. Thus clinicians need to use a wide range of behavioral observation and recording strategies to evaluate the individual and determine an initial and tentative diagnosis based on whether the individual's behavior meets specific criteria that make the person eligible for intervention services and supports. It is important in such cases to pursue several possibilities, including that the behavior, which is considered aberrant or disordered by some, is highly adaptable and responsive to very negative and deleterious environmental conditions. Good clinical judgment includes (a) incorporating broad assessment and evaluation strategies, (b) using standards with broad outcomes that relate to real-life application and that can be applied across age and environmental situations, (c) linking assessment to instruction or intervention, (d) involving the individual in ongoing self-assessment so as to teach self-determination skills, and (e) respecting self-determination.

Implementing Intervention Best Practices

Intervention techniques for people with mental retardation have changed significantly over the past four decades due in part to three phenomena: (a) research-based knowledge; (b) a new vision of people with mental retardation that encompasses equity, inclusion, empowerment, and personal well-being; and (c) the emergence of the ecological-behavioral perspective that stresses the functionality of behavior and the significant role of environments in a person's life (Schalock, Baker, & Croser, 2002). As a result of these three phenomena, intervention best practices are based today on the following four types of analyses, described more fully in chapter 6: descriptive analysis, functional analysis, ecological analysis, and outcome analysis.

Planning, Implementing, and Evaluating Individualized Supports

Since the 1980s the supports paradigm has focused our attention and efforts on obtaining valued personal outcomes for individuals with mental retardation and enhancing their functional capabilities and life situations. This focus is exemplified in the current emphasis on supported employment, supported living, and inclusive education. Supports are generally defined as "resources and strategies that aim to promote the development, education, interests, and personal well-being of a person and that enhance individual functioning" (Luckasson et al., 2002, p. 15). In reference to this clinical judgment strategy, three key aspects of the provision of supports are

- **support areas** such as: (a) life activities involving home living, community living, lifelong learning, employment, health and safety, social, and protection and advocacy; (b) exceptional medical conditions; and (c) exceptional behaviors (Thompson et al., 2002);

- **support functions** such as teaching, befriending, financial planning, employee assistance, behavioral support, in-home living assistance, community access and use, and health assistance (Luckasson et al., 2002, p. 148);

- **personal outcomes** related to independence, relationships, contributions, school and community participation, and personal well-being (Luckasson et al., 2002, p. 148).

Reflecting Cultural Competency and Linguistic Diversity

When an individual's language or culture is diverse, the evaluation team must take particular care to ensure that any assessment plan addresses the individual's abilities or disabilities, not simply the culture or language. This means that the team must create a plan that will (a) collect relevant information about the person and his or her home environment and/or language, (b) analyze the demands of the proposed environment and language, (c) complete a thorough social history that includes culture and language, (d) select suitable test instruments and outline necessary assessment modifications or accommodations, (e) provide an evaluator(s) who is sensitive to the person's language and culture, and (f) ensure that the assessment plan is implemented in a manner consistent with all legal and ethical guidelines. The individual's disability must not be overlooked, with the challenges being attributed to her or his minority culture or language rather than to the disability. Good clinical judgment and practice need to be employed to prevent this from happening.

Clinical Judgment Operational Actions

Each of the six clinical judgment strategies just discussed is operationalized through the actions summarized in Table 1.4. Each of these operational actions is used to provide the framework of the content of each chapter found in part 2. Note also that each action has a result related to the use of clinical judgment to communicate a decision or recommendation that answers the original question with a heightened degree of certainty and precision. The anticipated results of the six actions are listed in Table 1.5.

Table 1.4
Clinical Judgment Operational Actions

---

1. Clarify and state precisely the question(s) set before you.

2. Use a relevant framework for the statement of the question. The framework may be derived from statutory requirements, research-theoretical constructs, statements from authoritative organizations, or statements of public policy.

3. Conduct needed activities.

4. Analyze the data.

5. Develop a decision or recommendation.

6. Communicate the decision or recommendation.

Clinical Judgment Guidelines

One's operational actions need to be anchored within a broad set of clinical judgment guidelines based not just on research-based knowledge, professional standards, and professional codes of ethics, but also on the intent of clinical judgment, which is to facilitate good decision making based on experiences with the person, his or her environment, and data. The purpose of these guidelines, associated with each clinical judgment strategy (see chaps. 3–8), is to provide clinicians with a guide and standards. They can also be considered as a benchmark against which to evaluate clinical judgment practices to ensure that they are truly "best practices." Examples (see the appendix for a complete listing) include:

• Have a clear understanding of the question and the intended product.

• Use multiple data sources to answer the question.

• Take a wholistic approach to the person and obtain input from the person and significant others.

- Complete a thorough assessment of support needs and how they can best be met through the provision of individualized supports.
- Use standards with broad outcomes related to real-life application.
- Use assessment instruments that are sensitive to diversity, have norms that are based on diverse groups, and have acceptable psychometric properties.
- Ensure participation of necessary cultural informants or consultants and language accommodation.

Table 1.5

Clinical Judgment Actions and Results

Action: Clarify and state precisely the question set before you.
Results: establishes clear mutual understanding of all aspects of the inquiry

Action: Use a relevant framework for the statement of the question.
Results: identifies needed activities

Action: Conduct needed activities.
Results: provides data that increases certainty and precision

Action: Analyze the data.
Results: forms the basis for a decision or recommendation

Action: Develop a decision or recommendation.
Results: integrates the question with the relevant framework, the data and the analysis

Action: Communicate the decision or recommendation.
Results: transmits the decision or recommendation that answers the question placed before you

---

Summary

In summary, best practices in the field of mental retardation are based on research-based knowledge combined with professional ethics, professional standards, and clinical judgment. As discussed in this chapter, clinical judgment, as one of the four competencies comprising best practices, involves the use of strategies, actions, and guidelines. Clinical judgment is a special type of judgment rooted in a high level of clinical expertise and experience, and it emerges from extensive data. Over the past several decades, there has been considerable discussion of professional ethics and standards. Our analysis and synthesis of these ethical principles and professional standards (Table 1.1) have identified five core ethical principles (and corresponding professional standards): exhibits competence, exhibits professional and scientific responsibility, shows respect for people's rights and dignity, exhibits concern for others' welfare, and contributes to community and society. To date, there has not been a comparable development in the area of clinical judgment. Such is the purpose of this book. Although it is beyond the scope of this book to discuss research-based knowledge in depth, relevant aspects of this knowledge are incorporated into the clinical judgment strategies, operational actions, and guidelines discussed throughout the book.

As shown in Figure 1.1 clinical judgment plays a central but variable role in best practices. The more the situation reflects uncertainty, imprecision, ambiguity, and complexity, the greater is the need to use clinical judgment. Our intent in the next chapter is to show the relationship between critical thinking and clinical judgment. As we will see in the suggested process for clarifying the question at hand, the clinician must be clear about the question's focus, the critical thinking skills involved, and the form of the intended product. Only then can one begin to address the frequently complex decisions and recommendations that clinicians make regarding people with mental retardation.

CHAPTER 2

The Relationship Between Critical Thinking and Clinical Judgment

Overview

Just as good writing begins with a good outline, good clinical judgment is based on an initial clear and precise understanding of the question being asked. Here, for example, are some of the questions asked in cases that frame subsequent chapters:

- "Can you develop better programming for Ray based on positive behavior supports and valued outcomes?"
- "What is your recommendation regarding Judy being competent to take care of the child?"
- "Can you tell us—what was the impact of the burn and subsequent events on my client's quality of life?"
- "Does this defendant have mental retardation?"
- "Is this child eligible for special education services?"

Clinicians must clearly understand the question in order to exercise good clinical judgment. The clinician who does not understand the question runs a risk of attending to information that is irrelevant to the true question and even answering a question different from the one being asked. For example, if the question is "Is this person competent to parent the child?" but the clinician does not know the question or misunderstands the question as, "Does this individual have mental retardation?" the clinician's construction of an assessment strategy will likely be flawed, the clinician's answer will be unresponsive to the question, the clinician's judgment will not be precise or accurate, and the clinician's integrity will be compromised.

As discussed in the six chapters found in part 2, a competent answer to any of the above questions relies on the use of clinical judgment strategies, actions, and guidelines. At the outset, however, we note the foundational importance of the first operational action. It's too easy to overlook the most obvious task: to clarify and state precisely the question set before you. The purpose of this chapter is to discuss how that clarification is facilitated through understanding clearly the question's focus, critical thinking requirements, and intended or anticipated product. As shown in Figure 2.1, each of these components is defined operationally in terms of subcomponents, along with actions that the clinician needs to perform should the focus, requirement, and/or product need further clarification or precision. These actions indicate that the clinician may need to clarify questions in any number of ways, by asking for the question in writing, requesting further explanation, researching the specifics of the question, agreeing on definitions of particular terms, restating the question and confirming the restatement, consulting with others who understand the question better, and testing one's own understanding in other ways.

What Is the Question's Focus?

Typically, three types of questions are asked of clinicians: those related to diagnosis (e.g., "Does this person have mental retardation?"); classification (e.g., "Is this person whom we know has mental retardation competent to be a witness?" i.e., "How should we classify this individual with mental retardation—competent to be a witness or incompetent to be a witness?"); and planning supports (e.g., "What supports are required to assist this individual with mental retardation to be as competent as possible as a witness?"). In light of these three types of questions the following guidelines will facilitate answering yes to the question, "Is the focus clear?"

- If the question pertains to eligibility for services, benefits, or legal protections, the focus of the question is on *diagnosis*.

- If the question pertains to grouping for services, communication about selected characteristics, or the person's competency, the focus of the question is on *classification*. It is important to realize that "classification" is used for more than its historical purpose of grouping on the basis of levels of measured intelligence or limitations in adaptive behavior. Increasingly clinicians are asked binary (i.e., yes/no) classification questions regarding the person's competency to stand trial, parent, be one's own guardian, and/or retain custody.

- If the question pertains to enhancing personal outcomes, the focus of the question is on *planning supports*.

If you use these guidelines and the focus of the question still is not clear, request clarification and/or rephrasing of the question.

What Skills Does Answering the Question Require?

Once the focus is clear, one needs to clarify the critical thinking skills that are required to answer the question. Critical thinking is increasingly being recognized as the cognitive engine driving the processes of knowledge development and professional judgment in a wide variety of professional fields (American Philosophical Association, 1990; Facione & Facione, 1996).

Critical thinking skills are integral to understanding what skills are required to answer the question. As shown in Figure 2.1, answering the question may require one or more of the following skills: analysis, evaluation, inference, interpretation, and explanation. The definition of each requirement is presented in Table 2.1.

Purposeful clinical judgments rely on critical thinking skills to consider evidence, conceptualizations, methodologies, criteria, and contexts (Norris & Ennis, 1989). Thus in addition to the five requirements listed in Figure 2.1, critical thinking is a central

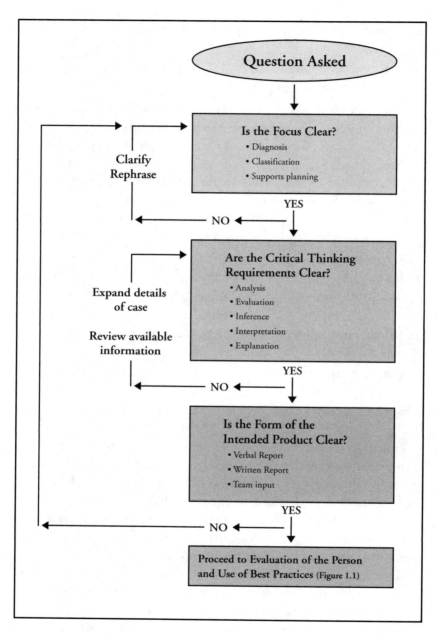

Figure 2.1. Process for clarifying the question at hand.

Table 2.1
Critical Thinking Skills Required to Answer the Question

Analysis: Examine the case, its elements, and its component parts; resolve the complexity of the case into simpler or more basic components or elements.

Evaluation: Determine the precision, accuracy, and integrity of available data through careful appraisal and study.

Inference: Form conclusions or recommendations on the basis of facts and/or premises. Standards against which to form a conclusion or recommendations include community presence, choice, competence, respect, community participation, satisfaction, and person-centeredness.

Interpretation: Integrate the available information in light of the individual's belief, judgment, or circumstance.

Explanation: Tell the meaning of the topic queried and present the explanation in understandable terms.

---

phenomenon in clinical judgment and also requires personal characteristics, such as the following (Facione & Facione, 1996):

- Truth seeking: having a courageous desire for the best knowledge in a context, even if such knowledge fails to support or undermines one's preconceptions, beliefs, or self-interests;
- Open-mindedness: showing tolerance toward divergent views and self-monitoring for possible bias;
- Analyticity: demanding the application of reason and evidence, being alert to problem situations, and being inclined to anticipate consequences;
- Systematicity: valuing organization and focusing on a reasoned

approached to complex problems;

- Self-confidence: trusting one's own reasoning skills;
- Inquisitiveness: being eager to acquire knowledge and to learn explanations even when applications of the knowledge are not immediately apparent;
- Maturity: being prudent in making, suspending, or revising judgment; being aware that multiple solutions may be acceptable and that reaching closure may be necessary even in the absence of complete knowledge.

What Is the Anticipated Product?

Yogi Berra reminded us of the importance of knowing where you are going ("or you might end up in the wrong place"). This is especially true in understanding clearly the question's intended or anticipated product: What form will the answer take? The product may vary from "communicating the clinician's decision to the involved individual or to the person asking the question" to "contributing to a team decision" to "preparing and presenting a formal report" to "participating in intervention and/or evaluation activities." These various products will be discussed more fully in reference to action steps involved in subsequent case studies. The key point is that if the clinician is unclear about the intended or anticipated product, he or she needs to ask for further clarification and explanation.

Conclusion and Guidelines

In conclusion, answering a question is one thing; being clear about what the question is really asking is quite another. Only when one truly understands the question's focus, along with required critical thinking skills and intended product can one determine the appropriate clinical judgment strategies to use. This chapter has emphasized that clarifying the question at hand requires an understanding of the question's focus, requirements, and intended product. Once these three factors and their associated guidelines (Table 2.2) are clearly understood, then one is ready to apply one or more clinical judgment strategies discussed in part 2. The first such strategy, conducting a thorough social history, forms the basis of the next chapter.

Table 2.2

Guidelines for Clarifying the Question at Hand

1. Be sure the focus of the question is clear: diagnosis, classification, or planning supports?

2. Understand the skill requirements inherent in answering the question: analysis, evaluation, inference, interpretation, and/or explanation?

3. Be clear on the intended product: What form will the answer take?

PART 2

Clinical Judgment Strategies

Although clinical judgment is always required, a number of situations necessitate a heightened reliance on clinical judgment to enhance decision making and facilitate best practices. These situations typically occur when:

- Formal assessment is less than optimal (e.g., unreliable, invalid, incomplete, inappropriate) and cannot be improved but, even so, is sufficient to provide a partial basis for pursuing clinical judgment.
- Complex medical or behavioral conditions are present that require multiple analyses.
- Legal restrictions significantly impact opportunities to assess the person.
- Cultural and/or linguistic diversity impact or affect the information needed for decisions.

These four situations typically require more than professional ethics, professional standards, and research-based knowledge; they require competent use of one or more of the following six clinical judgment strategies:

- Conduct a thorough social history.
- Align data and its collection to the critical question(s) at hand.
- Apply broad-based assessment strategies.
- Implement intervention best practices.
- Plan, implement, and evaluate individualized supports.

• Reflect cultural competence and linguistic diversity.

Each chapter in part 2 is based on an actual situation involving one of the authors who used one or more clinical judgment strategies to enhance the precision, accuracy, and integrity of the answer given to a particular question asked. In addition, the case study allows us to describe the operational actions taken and the relevant guidelines that provide a framework and standards for applying the respective strategy. In selecting the cases for inclusion, we have been sensitive to the multiple needs of clinicians who frequently face situations such as the four listed above. In that regard, the reader will find personal experiences related to the criminal justice system, legal system, intervention best practices, parental rights, quality of life, complex eligibility issues, and multicultural and linguistic challenges.

CHAPTER 3

Conducting a Thorough Social History: Does Darin Have Mental Retardation?

Overview

In this chapter we will look at the diagnostic case of Darin, a defendant in a criminal case. Compiling a thorough social history is always an important part of a diagnosis, but it is especially critical when a retroactive diagnosis is sought or when the stakes are high. In the case of most children today, compiling the social history is relatively easy because of mandated school records and the presence of the family. In the case of adults who have not previously had a diagnosis, however, compiling the thorough social history will demand more time and resources. If the stakes are very high, as in many legal and guardianship cases, considerable care and attention will be necessary to exercise good clinical judgment.

Since the early 1980s, the courts have become much more aware of the presence of defendants (and victims) with mental retardation in the criminal justice system. Recognizing the potential for unfairness, mistakes, and misunderstandings when a defendant or victim has mental retardation, courts began putting into place doctrines and procedures to improve the likelihood of justice when someone has mental retardation. For example, the U.S. Supreme Court in the case of *Atkins v. Virginia* (2002) ruled that it would violate the Eighth Amendment to the U.S. Constitution (the amendment that prohibits "cruel and unusual" punishment) to execute any individual with mental retardation. The Court recognized that individuals with this disability, as a group, have disabilities in reasoning, limitations in judgment, difficulties in control of impulses, and a lower level of moral culpability because of their cognitive disability.

The Supreme Court ruled in the *Atkins* case that the presence of mental retardation jeopardizes reliability and fairness of the death penalty process and undermines the strength of the procedural protections that might otherwise protect the defendant. For example, the Court ruled that mitigation doctrine alone is not sufficient protection, individuals with mental retardation are less able to assist their lawyers, are typically poor witnesses, have problems with demeanor that might interfere with their presentation to decision makers, are at risk for incorrect stereotypes about future dangerousness, and face special risk for wrongful execution.

In addition, the Court ruled that execution of defendants with mental retardation is not justified under two of the traditional justifications for the death penalty: retribution (because they have lower moral culpability) or deterrence (because they have lower ability to process information). Thus execution of defendants with mental retardation violates the Eighth Amendment, because the death penalty is excessive and disproportional based on state legislative actions and Supreme Court review.

The Court referenced the standard three components of the definition of mental retardation: significantly impaired intellectual ability, limitations in adaptive behavior, and presence before the age of 18. The Court referenced both the American Association on Mental Retardation (Luckasson et al., 1992) and the American Psychological Association (Jacobson & Mulick, 1996) definitions of mental retardation in footnote 3 of the *Atkins* (2002) opinion. The Court took a realistic view of people with the disability; it recognized that many people with mental retardation know right from wrong and are competent to stand trial. But the Court added that they have a diminished capacity to understand and process information, to communicate, to abstract from mistakes and learn from experience, to engage in logical reasoning, to control impulses, and to understand the reactions of others.

The Court in its decision anticipates the use of clinical judgment in the diagnosis of mental retardation. It is critical, therefore, to understand what clinical judgment is and who is entitled to use it. Certainly, clinical judgment is not mere unsubstantiated assumptions by anyone who happens to have an opinion; for example, an angry prison guard who concludes the defendant does not have mental retardation because the defendant beat him in a card game cannot legitimately claim that he is entitled to use clinical judgment or that his conclusion is the result of his clinical judgment.

The Supreme Court relied on the trend line of the actions of 18 death penalty states and the federal system that had outlawed the execution of defendants with mental retardation as evidence that prevailing standards have changed and modern Americans favor prohibition of execution of defendants with mental retardation. The diagnosis of mental retardation in an individual, always important, took on new gravity in the criminal justice system.

The Case of Darin

Darin is a 55-year-old African American who has been charged with a serious crime and is in jail awaiting trial. His appointed defense lawyer was initially very happy with Darin as a client because Darin is exceedingly polite and always agrees with everything the lawyer says. Darin is patient with all delays, thoughtful in asking about the health of the lawyer and her family, and does not complain, even about the jailhouse food.

The lawyer has become concerned, however, that Darin does not seem able to follow the lawyer's chronology of steps in the case and does not provide concrete information about anything including what happened during the incident. The lawyer thinks Darin might be incompetent to stand trial and perhaps even have mental retardation. The lawyer asked an investigator to search out the school records.

The skilled and hard-working investigator found several years of school records for Darin in the southern, rural community in which he grew up. There was no reference to special education or disability in the school records, nor any IQ scores or adaptive behavior assessments. When Darin entered school 49 years ago, it was a segregated Black school with limited resources and untrained and poorly paid teachers. This was around the time of the U.S. Supreme Court decision in *Brown v. Board of Education* (1954) but long before implementation of the desegregation decision. It also was decades before federal special education legislation reflected in the current Individuals With Disabilities Education Act of 2004 were enacted.

The lawyer has asked for an evaluation of mental retardation. A diagnosis of mental retardation requires the disability to have been present before the age of 18. Darin has never had an official diagnosis of mental retardation. To make a diagnosis, the clinician must assemble a thorough social history—to document whether a disability existed before the age of 18. Thus the primary critical thinking skills required included analysis, inference, interpretation, and explanation. The intended product was both a verbal and written report.

Clinical Judgment Actions

Clarify and State Precisely the Question Set Before You

In this case the lawyer is asking specifically whether Darin has mental retardation. According to this hypothetical, the lawyer has not yet asked the evaluator whether Darin is competent, although it appears likely that this may become a specific question in the future. If competence becomes an issue, it will be necessary to clarify with his lawyer "competence for what?" Competence is not a global conclusion but a particularized answer that depends on the legal question that was asked. Each type of competence (e.g., to stand trial, to be a witness, to make financial decisions) is a different legal question. Each type has different legal elements or components and thus requires a different evaluation tailored to those elements. An evaluation for each type of competence must specifically address the elements for the particular type of competence.

Use a Relevant Framework for the Statement of the Question

In the case of Darin, the immediate question asked by his lawyer is whether he has mental retardation. To develop a contextual framework for stating and answering the question, the clinician must understand the definition of mental retardation and its relevance to the criminal justice system.

The Supreme Court has referenced the American Association on Mental Retardation definition of mental retardation, with its three elements: (a) limitations in intellectual functioning, (b) limitations in adaptive behavior, and (c) presence of the disability before age 18 (Luckasson et al., 1992; 2002). The definition's relevance to the criminal justice system is reflected in three of its operative assumptions: (a) limitations in present functioning must be considered within the context of community environments typical of the individual's age peers and culture; (b) valid assessment considers cultural and linguistic diversity as well as differences in communication, sensory, motor, and behavioral factors; and (c) within an individual, limitations often coexist with strengths.

For individuals who are new to the criminal justice system or have been in the system for some time, making a diagnosis of mental retardation can be challenging due to one or more of the following situations: (a) the individual comes from a cultural and/or linguistic background that differs significantly from the mainstream; (b) earlier information is lacking or incomplete; (c) for security reasons, the individual's adaptive behavior functioning cannot be assessed consistently with the three operative assumptions listed above; (d) standardized assessment procedures are either not available or not appropriate, because the individual's status precludes their use and/or valid interpretation; (e) difficulties arise in selecting informants and validating informant observation; (f) direct observation of the individual's actual performance has been limited; and (g) difficulties arise when attempting to determine whether the age of onset criterion has been met.

Conduct Needed Activities

Darin does not currently have, nor has he ever had, a documented, official diagnosis of mental retardation. Does this mean that he does not have the disability? No, not necessarily. There is a difference between lack of documented diagnosis and lack of mental retardation. But because no one has been able to locate an official diagnosis from his childhood, Darin's evaluation will need to contain a thorough social history to determine whether a disability was present before age 18.

First, consider Darin's functioning as a child. Assuming that there are no intelligence tests or adaptive behavior assessments dating from his childhood, the evaluator will have to explore other types of documents and the memories of people familiar with Darin's childhood functioning to determine whether there was significantly impaired intellectual ability, limited adaptive behavior, and a disability manifested before age 18. Compiling a thorough social history that addresses the elements of mental retardation is essential.

When the stakes are high, perhaps life and death as they are in this case, the evaluator should work with a trained investigator who is an expert at obtaining life information. The investigator will interview the individual, investigate the individual's entire life, visit the area(s) where he was born and grew up, interview relatives and people who knew him as a child and youth, and assemble hundreds of documents including the following: birth certificate, birth and medical records, school records, social service records, church records, employment history, military records, mental health records, records on other family members, and all records of childhood and current functioning.

Analyze the Data

After completing this type of investigation and assembling these records, an evaluator should be able to form an opinion on whether the individual has mental retardation. Is his intellectual ability significantly impaired? Are there limitations in adaptive behavior? Were these present before the age of 18? Particularly when viewed in the context of the individual's measured current functioning, past functioning and diagnosis should become clear even when there is not "official" diagnosis from childhood.

Develop a Decision or Recommendation

In Darin's case the investigation reaffirmed the poverty and isolation of his childhood community as well as the lack of available educational services. The investigation also revealed limited maternal prenatal care, a difficult birth, a history of school failures, documented head injuries, and family and neighbor memories of how "slow" Darin was. When viewed in the context of Darin's current significantly impaired intellectual functioning and limited adaptive behavior as measured by testing, the evaluator concluded that Darin has mental retardation that was present since childhood. This was reported to the lawyer who proceeded with decisions about any further questions, such as competence to stand trial, that might require additional evaluations.

Communicate the Decision or Recommendation

The evaluator should communicate his decision and recommendation to the lawyer and wait for further instructions. The evaluator should pay particular attention to the form the communication should take. Because of the nature of legal proceedings, the evaluator may be asked for a privileged recommendation protected by attorney-client confidentiality or for recommendations that might become part of the record of the case. The evaluator should not assume that one form fits all; if the request is unclear, the evaluator should clarify with the lawyer what form the recommendation should take. Later an evaluator may be asked to provide recommendations in other forms, such as depositions or court testimony.

Summary and Guidelines

Compiling a thorough social history is always an important part of a diagnosis, but it is especially critical when a retroactive diagnosis is sought or when the stakes are high. In the case of most children today, this is generally relatively easy because of school mandates for special education, contemporary records, and the presence in the immediate environment of family and other people who know the child and the child's functioning. In the case of adults who have not previously had a diagnosis, however, compiling the thorough social history will demand more time and resources. If the stakes are very high, for example the question of whether the Constitution permits the person to be eligible for execution, considerable care and attention will be necessary to exercise clinical judgment. Key guidelines to assist this effort are summarized in Table 3.1.

Table 3.1
Guidelines for Conducting a Social History

1. Clarify any legal question and the form the recommendations should take.

2. Be aware of current legal findings and definitions.

3. Investigate, collect, and organize all relevant information about the person's life including stages, trajectory, development, functioning, relationships, and family.

4. Explore the possible reasons for differences in data, including (a) poorly trained examiner, (b) improper generalization of test scores administered for other purposes, (c) improper selection of tests, (d) neglect of consideration of standard error of measurement, (e) mistakes in scoring, (f) administrations of the same test too close in time, (g) different editions of the same test and resultant Flynn effects, (h) bias, and (i) behavioral differences in the individual.

5. Develop contemporary assessment, if indicated, in order to show changes in functioning over the life span.

CHAPTER 4

Aligning Data and Its Collection to the Critical Questions Asked: The Case of Matt

Overview

The attorney from Denver was quite matter of fact when he called and said, "This case may stretch your creativity and skills. We are representing a client who was burned severely in a bathtub accident at this group home, and we are approaching the case from a quality-of-life perspective. By the way, his level of intellectual functioning is well within the profound range. Can you tell us—what was the impact of the burn and subsequent events on the quality of my client's life?"

The young man's name was Matt. His case presented at least four challenges related to the second clinical judgment strategy: aligning data and its collection to the critical questions asked. First, can the concept of quality of life be used for forensic purposes, given that the concept provides a conceptual model to evaluate the effects of injury or trauma (Williams & Murphy, 2000)? Second, how does one operationalize the concept of quality of life to measure the impact of a trauma or injury on the person's assessed quality of life? Third, how does one evaluate the quality of life of someone like Matt whose cognitive and language skills are limited? And fourth, how can all this be done within the context of an adversarial process? The remainder of this chapter is devoted to answering those four questions and coming to a decision and recommendation that answers the attorney's question, "What was the impact of the burn and subsequent events on Matt's quality of life?" The focus in answering the question was on overcoming some of the stereotypes associated with classification systems and on developing an individualized support plan. The critical thinking skills centered around analysis, evaluation, inference, and explanation. The intended product was a written report.

Matt and His Trauma

Based on a thorough social history and personal observation and using nontraditional assessment strategies, the following five aspects of Matt's life and experiences prior to and immediately after the burn incident were clear.

- Matt should not be considered a person with profound retardation, with no ability to learn or change. He should rather be considered within the broader context of the two important factors regarding people such as Matt: (a) specific adaptive limitations often coexist with strengths in other adaptive skills or personal capabilities; and (b) with appropriate supports over a sustained period, the life functioning of the person will generally improve (Luckasson et al., 2002).

- Throughout his life and up until the time of the burn incident, Matt demonstrated the potential for growth, adaptation, development, and learning—the potential to live a more fulfilling life. This potential (as reported in school and adult-service-provider records) is reflected in, for example, his adjusting to new situations, speaking four words, feeding himself with minimum assistance, making progress on a toilet training program, making eye contact, cooperating with staff, responding to his name, finding and retrieving materials of interest from cupboards, loving to run around a track, occupying himself with keys and other bright objects, indicating his wants/needs by standing near the desired object, enjoying participating in community-based activities, sitting for a short time listening to stories or music, and beginning to use a communication/picture board to help with communication.

- The care and treatment or training Matt received was meant to enhance his quality of life, including fulfillment. Although Matt's quality of life (as reported by his mother and residential staff) was enhanced generally, it improved to different degrees in differing domains. For example, he tended to show more growth and development in the areas of motor functioning (e.g., running and walking), self-help skills (e.g., self-feeding and assisting with dressing), and emotional bonding and relating to others than he did in expressive language and cognitive skills.

- Immediately prior to the burn incident, Matt was adjusting well to a community living arrangement and developing new skills and behaviors.

- The burn incident contributed significant and additional stressors to Matt's life, including: the actual burn; the burn treatment itself and the apparent tachycardia, evident in the hospital following the burn; the use of restraints while in the hospital following the burn; the naso-gastric (NG) tube inserted and used since the incident; the loss of his possessions when he was removed from his residence; the additional allergic reactions that became apparent in the hospital; and his placement following release from the hospital into a very institutional, maintenance facility rather than a home in which his rehabilitation needs could be met.

Clinical Judgment Actions

Clarify and State Precisely the Question Set Before You

It took a number of conference calls to agree on what the actual question was and what was the intended product. It became very apparent during these sessions that different disciplines (e.g., law and psychology) approach the same concept from very different perspectives. Legal definitions and the processes involved in aggregating data (and "evidence") are frequently different from the operational definitions and processes psychologists employ to study a phenomenon such as quality of life. Over time, however, agreement was reached on how quality of life would be defined and measured, what processes would be used to determine the impact of the burn experience, and what format the data would need to be aggregated into (and presented to the court) to both answer the question and meet the legal requirements of the litigation process.

Use a Relevant Framework for the Statement of the Question

To develop a relevant framework for stating and answering the question, one often needs a clear understanding of knowledge based on research. This was definitely the case with Matt; because quality of life is still an emerging field, one must be aware of how it is currently being conceptualized and measured. The question dealing with the impact of the burn and subsequent events on Matt's quality of life required that the evaluator understand not only what is meant by quality of life, but also how one measures it in a preincident-postincident way.

There is now good agreement based on the international quality-of-life literature that a life of quality (for individuals with mental retardation as with others) is composed of eight core domains. These eight domains, along with their three most common behavioral indicators are as follows:

- Emotional well-being: contentment, self-concept, freedom from stress
- Interpersonal relations: interactions, relationships, supports (emotional, physical, financial, feedback)
- Material well-being: financial status, employment, housing
- Personal development: education, personal competence, performance
- Physical well-being: health, activities of daily living, leisure
- Self-determination: autonomy/personal control, goals and personal values, choices
- Social inclusion: community integration and participation, community roles, social supports

- Rights: human (respect, dignity, equality), legal (citizenship, access, due process). (Schalock & Verdugo, 2002, pp. 184–187)

The challenge in Matt's case was to develop behavioral indicators that would reflect his cognitive, language, and physical limitations *and* assess the quality-of-life indicators listed above for each domain. To do this we developed interview questions to be asked of those who best knew Matt and behavioral indicators to be evaluated by observation. These questions and indicators are summarized in Table 4.1.

Significantly, the data sets summarized in Table 4.1 not only clearly align the question asked to needed information, but they also indicate that nontraditional assessment strategies will be required to obtain that information. How this was done is described in the next clinical judgment action.

Conduct Needed Activities

To determine that something (such as the burn incident and subsequent events) has had an impact, one must demonstrate significant pre-post differences in the phenomenon being observed (in this case, Matt's quality of life). Two activities were conducted to determine if there was an impact. The first was to use Table 4.1 to organize and aggregate Matt's preaccident behavioral indicators into the respective quality-of-life domains based on answers to questions asked of his mother and residential staff and observation conducted by the author. The results are shown in the center column of Table 4.2.

The second activity involved observing Matt following the incident and his hospital stay plus asking the same questions (Table 4.1) of his mother and residential staff, but this time the questions referred to his postaccident status. This information is summarized in the right-hand column of Table 4.2.

Table 4.1

Interview Questions and Behavioral Indicators Used to Assess Matt's Quality of Life

Questions to be asked of family and residential staff regarding preincident behaviors and responses. (Reword questions into past tense.) Questions also to be asked about postincident behaviors and responses. (Ask questions in present tense.) Ask respondents to give examples rather than answering questions with a simple yes or no.

Emotional well-being: How does Matt respond to pain? How does he express pleasure and contentment? How does he behave when afraid? Any evidence of earlier bathing incidents?

Interpersonal relations: What is the range of Matt's vocalizations? Any indication of a pattern of potential friendships with other residents or staff? How does Matt show affection?

Material well-being: What are Matt's most preferred possessions? How does he act when his name is called, (b) someone gets close to him, and (c) a preferred object is removed?

Personal development: What is the most complicated task Matt can complete? What is the range of exhibited positive behaviors? What is the range of exhibited challenging (negative) behaviors?

Physical well-being: What is his sleep behavior? What is your perception of his ability to see, hear, taste, walk, run?

Self-determination: What is the range of Matt's likes and dislikes? How does he express what he needs and wants? How does he express his likes and dislikes?

Social inclusion: What are Matt's preferred indoor and outdoor activities with other people? How does he act around the various people around him?

Rights: Does Matt defend or protect what he feels is his? Is he modest or self-conscious about having his clothes removed or being without clothes in front of others?

Table 4.2 Pre- and Post-Incident Behavioral Quality-of-Life-Related Indicators		
Domain	**Preincident Status**	**Postincident Status**
Emotional well-being	alert, giggles, laughs, smiles appropriately	increased fear and avoidant responses
Interpersonal relations	involvement with mother and brother, curious and explores, cooperates with staff	no apparent change
Material well-being	self-abuse regarding threat to space, oriented to name, demonstrates object permanence	no apparent change
Personal development	follows 1-step commands, toilet trained, attends, communicates with simple gestures, partially self-feeding	follows directions less, reduced self-help and prevocational skills
Physical well-being	good nutritional status, motor skills intact, no sleep disturbance, range of motion	NG tube flushed 3 times a day, reduced gross motor skills
Self-determination	communication, gestures, makes needs known, seeks out favorite people, dislikes having hair combed	no apparent change
Social inclusion	generally passive in response to others, but enjoys being around others, likes going outside	reduced community integration, reduced community participation
Rights	ownership and personal autonomy	reduced opportunity to exercise rights

Analyze the Data

Once the data were aggregated as shown in Table 4.2, its analysis was straightforward. Although no statistical tests were conducted (due to the data being based on interviews and personal observation), the trend is very apparent in the table: the incident and subsequent events had significant and direct negative impacts on five (emotional well-being, personal development, physical well-being, social inclusion, and rights) of the eight quality-of-life domains.

Develop a Decision or Recommendation

As mentioned throughout the text, the three criteria of good clinical judgment are its being systematic (i.e., organized, sequential, and logical), formal (i.e., explicit and reasoned), and transparent (i.e., apparent and communicated clearly). Meeting these three criteria allowed the clinician to state with increased certainty and precision the following:

- The incident and subsequent events had significant and direct negative impacts on five quality-of-life domains: emotional well-being, personal development, physical well-being, social inclusion, and rights.
- The incident also had indirect and potentially negative impacts on all of the other three quality-of-life domains. For example, interpersonal relations are affected due to the increased fear and avoidant responses and the reduced opportunity for modeling due to the new institutional placement; self-determination and material well-being are affected due to reduced choices and options, reduced self-help skills, and reduced prevocational skills.

Communicate the Decision or Recommendation

Following receipt of the above written decision-recommendation, the clinician involved in Matt's case was asked to suggest a number of remedies that could be implemented that would have a high probability of enhancing the quality of Matt's life. These suggested remedies that became part of the final written report are listed below, aggregated according to the respective quality-of-life core domain.

- emotional well-being: emotional bonding and desensitization training
- interpersonal relations: teaching trust through bonded family and staff; housemate to establish parallel play and peer interaction
- material well-being: homelike environment that would provide safe and personal space; personal possessions
- personal development: active teaching (e.g., attending skills, compliance behavior, fine motor skills); channel his interests and curiosity with highly preferred activities
- physical well-being: medical nursing including seizure control; proper nutrition, especially hydration; occupational and physical therapy
- self-determination: communication system; choice and opportunities
- social inclusion: community outings and activities
- rights: *Olmstead* (1999) ruling regarding the right to live in the community and *Wyatt v. Stickney* (1972) regarding right to active treatment

Summary and Guidelines

Questions are often easy to ask but difficult to answer. This was especially true of Matt's case, because of the significant challenges it presented. Moreover, the question asked about the impact of the burn on Matt's quality of life was not a question that could be answered on the basis of only research-based knowledge, only professional ethics, or only professional standards. Thus this second clinical judgment strategy reflects a growing need that clinicians will undoubtedly face: the request to expand their skills in the techniques and strategies they use to align data and its collection to critical questions asked. This clinical strategy is very consistent with the current emphasis on practice-based evidence that represents the contributions of practitioners who use research methodologies to examine the quality of their clinical practice and service provision

(Newman, Kellett, & Beail, 2003). Five guidelines that are essential to aligning data to the question asked and providing practice-based evidence are summarized in Table 4.3.

Table 4.3

Guidelines for Aligning Data and Its Collection to the Critical Questions Asked

---

1. Understand clearly what question is being asked and what data will be required to answer it.

2. Establish one's competence to pursue the clinical judgment actions that are required.

3. Use research-based knowledge to incorporate currently available measures and strategies or use professional standards to develop needed data-collection techniques.

4. Use multiple data sources (e.g., personal appraisal or functional assessment) to obtain the necessary data.

5. Show clearly that the obtained data is aligned with the critical question(s) asked.

CHAPTER 5

Broad-Based Assessment Strategies: Is Carmen Eligible for Special Education Services?

Overview

Broad-based assessment strategies permit a full picture of an individual's functioning; they are the means for the systematic collection of relevant data about a person's disabilities and abilities. The purpose of broad assessment strategies is to develop and test one or more hypotheses about diagnosis and the provision of supports. The testing of hypotheses regarding a potential diagnosis should be systematic and based on logical, disciplined inquiry and best practices. For example, the 2002 American Association on Mental Retardation definition of mental retardation includes an important assumption of broad assessment in that, "limitations in present functioning must be considered within the context of community environments typical of the individual's age peers and culture" (Luckasson et al., p. 1).

The purpose of broad assessment strategies is to answer the question(s) set before the clinician within the strategies, actions, and guidelines of clinical judgment. Typically, questions will be related to the person's diagnosis and/or the development of individualized support systems. A broad-based assessment needs to be initiated and directed by a clinician, following the ethical principles and professional standards summarized in Table 1.1. In the assessment, the human and legal rights of the individual must be respected, with the ultimate goal of the process being the enhancement of the individual's personal well-being (Schalock, 2001). These introductory comments are important to keep in mind as you consider the circumstances of Carmen.

The Case of Carmen

For years Carmen lived mostly on the streets with her father after her paternal grandmother died when Carmen was a toddler. Her father had a significant mental illness that became more severe after the death of his own mother; he believed that if Carmen went to school, bad things would happen to them. Carmen cooperated with her father's beliefs; she feared that if she reported the situation to any authorities, she and her father would be separated. Carmen and her father, through a variety of strategies, together successfully evaded detection by most authorities. Carmen felt that she could not risk separation, because her father needed her to care for him when he was sick. But when Carmen was 10 her father died. Carmen was ill, and she determined that she could not safely continue alone and would have to seek help from some authorities. After several attempted attacks, from which she narrowly escaped, she reluctantly asked for help from a police officer who looked kind.

Many complications and delays later, Carmen was placed with a foster family and enrolled in the neighborhood elementary school. She cannot read or write, is unfamiliar with and resistant to expected hygiene routines, does not seem to sleep, cries most of the night, has poor to no verbal communication, and bites when either foster parent tries to comfort her.

The foster parents and her teacher believe she needs special education supports. Is she eligible for special education services? The focus of the question was diagnosis. Due to Carmen's behavioral impairment, the critical thinking skills required involved analysis, evaluation, inference, and interpretation. The intended product was both team input and a written report regarding an initial diagnosis and the formulation of an individualized support plan.

Clinical Judgment Actions

Clarify and State Precisely the Question(s) Set Before You

The foster parents and teacher clarified and stated precisely the question: Is Carmen eligible for special education services? As discussed in subsequent sections, answering this question required not just the use of broad-based assessment strategies, but also the use of considerable systematic behavioral observations in multiple settings.

Use a Relevant Framework for the Statement of the Question

The school psychologist realized that because of Carmen's lack of verbal communication, present emotional distress, and challenging behaviors, formal testing was inappropriate at this early point.

During the initial school-assistance meeting that involved Carmen, her foster parents, her general education teacher, a special education teacher, and psychologist, the team reviewed the criteria for the potentially applicable diagnoses: mental retardation, learning disability, and emotional disturbance. Based on her history, current functioning, and current behaviors, the team decided that the most appropriate working diagnosis was emotional disturbance. Testing this diagnostic hypothesis required familiarity with the characteristics of children with this disorder and a variety of assessment strategies that would explore whether these characteristics existed in Carmen's functioning, thereby justifying the diagnosis of an emotional disturbance. The strategies used will be discussed in the following action step ("conduct needed activities").

The Individuals With Disabilities Education Act (2004) defines emotional disturbance:

> (i) The term means a condition exhibiting one or more of the following characteristics over a long time and to a marked degree that adversely affects a student's educational performance: (a) an inability to learn that cannot be explained by intellectual, sensory, or health factors; (b) an inability to build or maintain satisfactory interpersonal relationships with peers or teachers; (c) inappropriate types of behavior

or feelings under normal circumstances; (d) a general pervasive mood of unhappiness or depression; and (e) a tendency to develop physical symptoms or fears associated with personal or school problems.

(ii) The term includes schizophrenia. The term does not apply to children who are socially maladjusted, unless it is determined that they have an emotional disturbance. (34 CFR § 300.7(c)(4))

An alternative definition has been proposed that should also be considered by the assessment team. The National Joint Committee on Learning Disabilities and the Mental Health and Special Education Coalition (McIntyre & Forness, 1996) developed the following definition and criteria for children with an emotional or behavioral disorder:

1. The term emotional or behavioral disorder means a disability that is: (a) characterized by behavioral or emotional responses in school programs so different from appropriate age, cultural, or ethnic norms that the responses adversely affect educational performance, including academic, social, vocational, or personal skills; (b) more than a temporary, expected response to stressful events in the environment; (c) consistently exhibited in two different settings, at least one of which is school-related; and (d) unresponsive to direct intervention applied in general education, or the condition of a child such that general education interventions would be insufficient.

2. The term includes such a disability that co-exists with other disabilities.

3. The term includes schizophrenic disorder, affective disorder, anxiety disorder, or other sustained disorder of conduct or adjustment, affecting a child if the disorder affects educational performance. (pp. 6–7)

Due to the complexity of Carmen's current cognitive and behavioral limitations, both of these definitions were used as a framework for conducting the following diagnostic activities.

Conduct Needed Activities

The diagnostic approach the clinician used was based on the principle that a primary purpose of a diagnosis is intervention planning. Hence, two behavioral observation strategies were used to (a) confirm the presence of the criteria used for establishing an initial diagnosis of emotional disturbance (as summarized in the previous section) with consequent eligibility and (b) provide the basis of schoolwide, classroom, and home-based individualized intervention and supports planning.

The first activity was to develop a rating scale that would be used by Carmen, the teacher, an educational assistant, and the foster parents to evaluate the pattern of each of Carmen's challenging behavior areas: hygiene routine, sleep pattern, and biting others. The rating scale that was completed daily for one month was formatted as follows:

Challenging Behavior	Rating
Hygiene routine	3 = does independently
	2 = does with assistance
	1 = does not do or resists
Sleep pattern	3 = Uninterrupted sleep for most of night
	2 = Disturbed sleep half of night (3–4 hr)
	1 = Disturbed sleep most of night (4+ hr)
Abuse of others	3 = Seldom bites
	2 = Bites 3–4 times per day
	1 = Bites 5 or more times per day

Carmen also was asked to complete the above recording sheet as part of her "homework assignment." To facilitate her participation, an iconic response format permitted her to circle the respective option for each of the three challenging behaviors. The frequency of these behaviors could then be used to determine whether her behavior impairment was: (a) a significant limitation, compared to her classmates; (b) more than temporary; and (c) exhibited at home as well as at school (i.e., across two environments).

The second activity was to have the teacher and foster mother complete an antecedent-behavior-consequence (ABC) analysis regarding Carmen's three challenging behaviors and three positive behaviors related to attempted verbalizations, social involvement, and cooperation. The overarching principle here is that one always looks for strengths as well as evaluates weaknesses or limitations. The format for this activity was a simple one-page sheet to be completed daily for 30 days based on the following parameters:

Behavior: A listing of the above-referenced three challenging and three positive behaviors.

Antecedent: For each occurrence of the listed behavior, the observer notes what preceded the behavior (e.g., a request? a frustrating occurrence? was she attempting to communicate? was Carmen interacting with another person?).

Consequence: The observer notes the function the behavior serves Carmen. Here the focus is on the results to Carmen when she exhibits the behavior. Two consequences are possible: (a) She receives positive reinforcement that results in attention or positive consequences, or (b) she experiences negative reinforcement that results in removing Carmen from something she perceives as unpleasant or allows her to avoid something unpleasant.

The ABC analysis can be used by the clinician to determine some of the potential causes of Carmen's challenging behaviors, potential positive behaviors on which to base positive behavioral support programs, and potential responsiveness to school and home-based intervention and individualized supports.

Analyze the Data

A clinician would not make a definitive diagnosis based on the data resulting from the rating scale and ABC analysis summarized above. However, until Carmen's behavior is stabilized, using a standard instrument to validly assess her strengths and limitations is highly improbable. Thus, in Carmen's case, as with many others like Carmen, the clinician is required to make an initial tentative diagnosis and in that process be guided by the clinical judgment guidelines summarized later in Table 5.1. In Carmen's case, both the rating scale and ABC analysis data suggested strongly that she met the definitional criteria of emotional disturbance and thus would be eligible for special education services in her state.

Develop a Decision or Recommendation

Clearly, evaluation of Carmen is going to be an ongoing process with several possible diagnoses being explored. Any early diagnosis must be considered tentative, because she seems to show strong signs of several types of disabilities. The assessment team must also be mindful, however, of the possibility that Carmen's serious limitations are the result of lack of schooling and unstable life, and that her behaviors were adaptive under those extraordinary circumstances. Individuals living as the "forgotten generation" (Tymchuk, Lakin, & Luckasson, 2001) present complex challenges in diagnosis and services.

Communicate the Decision or Recommendation

The primary purposes of a diagnosis are for eligibility (if necessary) and for intervention planning. Hence there must be an immediate recommendation for an individualized plan of supports that addresses the complex issues raised in Carmen's life, including individualized academic instruction, behavioral intervention, and supports.

Summary and Guidelines

In summary, the lives of many individuals referred for evaluation are complex. Evaluations of their disabilities must take into account this complexity by using broad-based assessment strategies. At the initial stages, these evaluations should contain elements of tentativeness and include continual reevaluation of diagnostic hypotheses. But the assessment must also be linked to the individual's needs for supports to improve learning, emotional status, and daily functioning while the diagnostic process continues.

As reflected in this chapter, clinical judgment requires flexibility and openness to broad-based assessment strategies and a variety of diagnostic hypotheses. As we see in the assessment of Carmen, a person's behavior or emotional status may temporarily interfere with formal testing even as a diagnosis for eligibility must be made in order to deliver critical services. The clinician is therefore required to use systematic behavioral observation techniques and recording strategies in multiple environments and obtain critical input from key informants including the individual. The assessment team must attempt to garner input from the person, because of the tremendous value contributed by the individual.

Flexibility and openness in a broad assessment strategy require that the clinician consider components of a variety of disabling conditions and not turn automatically to a preordained protocol to attempt to answer the question(s) asked. The clinician must hold a sufficient number of diagnostic possibilities in mind while pursuing the broad assessment strategies suggested in this chapter. Guidelines to facilitate that process are summarized in Table 5.1.

Table 5.1
Broad-Based Assessment Guidelines

1. Incorporate a broad evaluative strategy.

2. Use standards with broad outcomes that relate to real-life application and can be applied across age and situations; be flexible enough that you look at the real-life application respecting the person and demands.

3. Link assessment to instruction or intervention.

4. Involve the individual in self-assessment on a regular basis.

5. Assessments may be refined as the person's condition, status, or functioning changes.

CHAPTER 6

Intervention Best Practices: The Case of Ray

Overview

Intervention techniques for people with mental retardation have changed significantly over the past four decades. New trends have included behavior modification, contingency management, overcorrection, satiation, token economies, aversive techniques, poly pharmacy, environmental modification, positive behavior supports, self-contained classrooms, behavior-shaping units, and one or more approaches to psychotherapy and counseling.

At the same time, we have experienced two significant shifts in our thinking. One is a new vision of people with mental retardation—a vision that encompasses equity, inclusion, empowerment, and personal well-being (Luckasson et al., 2002). The other is the ecological-behavioral perspective that stresses the functionality of behavior and the significant role that environments play in either the disabling or the enhanced performance process (World Health Organization, 2001).

These two changes have had a tremendous impact on intervention best practices. No longer do we think only about the individual's behavior in isolation. Increasingly we realize that intervention best practices are characterized by using four types of analyses:

- **Descriptive analysis** that focuses on the individual's strengths and limitations. It includes diagnostic evaluations and nontraditional assessments and leads to education and rehabilitation programs and therapeutic interventions. It answers the question, "Who is this person from a descriptive perspective?"

- **Functional analysis** that focuses on behavior and its communicative intent. It includes antecedent-behavior-consequence (ABC) analysis and the communicative intent of behavior. It leads to positive behavior support programs and answers the question, "What does the behavior tell us?"

- **Ecological analysis** that focuses on the person's interaction with his or her environment. It includes an analysis of the discrepancy between the person's capabilities and the environment's demands. It leads to the use of prosthetics, environmental accommodation or adaptation, and assistive technology. It answers the question, "How can environments be used to enhance personal development and personal well-being?"

- **Outcome analysis** that focuses on desired person-referenced outcomes including those related to the eight quality-of-life domains (emotional well-being, interpersonal relations, material well-being, personal development, physical well-being, self-determination, social inclusion, and rights). It includes person-centered planning and the supports paradigm. It leads to organizational or staff alignment and outcomes-based evaluation. It answers the question, "Have personal goals and dreams been achieved?"

The clinical judgment shown in the following case of Ray demonstrates clearly how the results of these four types of analyses can be integrated into a positive behavior support plan that reflects the fourth clinical judgment strategy (i.e., implementing intervention best practices) and clinical actions and guidelines associated with it.

The Case of Ray

Involvement with Ray began with a call from a state protection and advocacy staff member. The state Department of Developmental Disabilities and the state protection and advocacy office were at an impasse about Ray, currently receiving services in a state-operated facility. The situation involved potential litigation regarding the apparent lack of rehabilitation programming and Ray's physical and psychological condition. The state's attorney general's office was also involved and suggested that the two groups "find someone you both can work with and have that person work with you to develop better programming for Ray."

At various times, reports of Ray's positive behaviors included descriptors such as cheerful, social, gregarious, outgoing, active, strongly motivated, communicative, a willing learner with a wide variety of interests, and one who has pride in doing things well. Historically, Ray exhibited a wide-range of challenging behaviors that included agitation, aggression, property destruction, self-induced vomiting, self-injurious behavior (SIB), and inappropriate attention getting. Ray's challenging behaviors, in conjunction with various medical and psychiatric problems, have resulted in at least eight residential moves over the past 15 years. He is currently living in a state-operated community residence with three other service recipients.

The case demonstrates that the question(s) asked can pertain to a team as well as an individual and that the skills involved include not only the critical thinking skills summarized in Table 2.1, but also personal characteristics of the clinician, such as truth seeking, open-mindedness, self-confidence, and maturity. The intended product included both written reports and input to Ray's team.

Clinical Judgment Actions

Clarify and State Precisely the Question Set Before You

The initial question was "Are you interested in and available for consultation?" The second question was "Can you help?" Neither question provided much guidance as to what was really needed. It took several conference calls and observation sessions with Ray to ferret out the real question: "Can you help us resolve the current impasse by working with all parties and by developing a credible and acceptable approach to Ray's behavioral programming?" The first part of the question required a yes or no answer; the second required the critical thinking skills related to analysis, evaluation, inference, interpretation, and definitely explanation.

Use a Relevant Framework for the Statement of the Question

The framework for answering the question requires multiple strategies, because of Ray's complex medical and behavioral conditions. The primary clinical judgment strategy needed in this case was to implement and evaluate intervention best practices. Three other clinical judgment strategies were tangentially involved. In the process of conducting the needed activities, it was necessary to apply broad-based assessment strategies (as part of the four types of analyses described earlier), develop a positive behavior support plan (which is a type of individualized support), and align data and its collection to the critical question asked. Answering the question (as eventually understood) asked by the attorney general's office and the other stakeholders involved these four strategies as well as integrating considerable data from multiple sources into a concerted and clearly expressed plan that focused on positive techniques and opportunities to enhance positive behaviors and decrease problem behaviors.

Conduct Needed Activities

The needed activities involved undertaking four types of analyses. Each of the four types of analyses was based on personal observation of Ray and conversations with him, record review, and face-to-face sessions with Ray's mother, residential staff, and case manager. Specific results of these analyses are as follows:

- **Descriptive analysis:** The above-mentioned people described Ray's strengths as including being determined or strong willed, social, communicative, and motivated. His three principal challenging behaviors were identified as agitation, SIB, and inappropriate attention getting. His current medications are Trileptal (750 mg/ day) and Baclofen (100 mg/day).

- **Functional analysis:** Each of the three challenging behaviors was analyzed in regard to its antecedents and hypothesized functions. For example, the antecedents for agitation were identified to be frustration, disappointment, and discomfort, with the hypothesized functions being to control staff or the environment, to express anger, and/or to regulate emotion. For SIB, the antecedents included agitation or frustration, staff attending to others, and/or discomfort. The hypothesized functions were to discharge feelings of anger, to get attention, to experience disappointment with self, and/or to displace pain. For inappropriate attention getting, the antecedents were wanting attention, unpredictability, loss of control, and/or getting an undesired response. The hypothesized functions of these behaviors included reducing feelings of boredom, controlling his environment, and/or communication.

- **Ecological analysis:** An extensive discussion with the abovementioned people indicated the need to reduce the "mismatch" between Ray and his environment by: focusing on how his wheelchair could be adapted to better meet his current need; adding bathroom supports and grab bars; using adaptive dishes and silverware; introducing communication devices such as computer-generated voice box or a functional communication board; adding a lift to the van; having Ray's vision evaluated; and providing grief therapy and other forms of family therapy to deal with family issues.

- **Outcome analysis:** Three behaviors (self-help skills, purposive at-home activities, and community activities) were selected because they were meaningful to Ray and his future. In the course of face-to-face discussions with residential staff, the following aspects of all three behaviors were determined: their definitions (with examples), activities used to develop the skills, procedures to use, necessary environmental adaptations, and positive consequences to Ray.

Analyze the Data

Two skills associated with this clinical judgment action were used: inductive and deductive reasoning and person-centered planning concepts. The data analyzed were those resulting from the four best-practice analyses described above. The analysis included organizing the data into a coherent program that could be easily communicated and used by the respective stakeholders, resolving the impasse, and making a difference in Ray's life. To accomplish these purposes we developed a positive behavior support plan, summarized in Table 6.1.

Develop a Decision or Recommendation

This fifth clinical judgment action step involved developing a positive behavior support program that would meet the three criteria of good clinical judgment: systematic, formal, and transparent. The parameters of that plan are summarized in Table 6.1.

Communicate the Decision or Recommendation

It is important to point out that the implementation and evaluation of intervention best practices require at least the following:

- clear delineation of target behaviors
- clear operational definitions
- easy-to-understand and -use recording forms
- frequent summary and analysis of the outcomes or data
- a report back to the principal stakeholders
- any changes made to the intervention, if necessary, based on data

The positive behavior support plan for Ray was accepted by all the stakeholders and implemented through a series of staff training sessions. Monthly graphs of the accelerated and decelerated behaviors are shared with all stakeholders and serve as the basis for changes in Ray's program.

Summary and Guidelines

This clinical judgment strategy—implement intervention best practices—is probably not found in any textbook. Each separate analysis—descriptive, functional, ecological, and outcome—is described in many texts, but putting these four analyses into one integrated and well-formatted process reflects both the clinical judgment strategy and clinical and behavioral best practices. Ray is a different person today and feels better about himself. He, along with his family, sees purpose to and change in his life. Ray often uses the word *happy*. The protection and advocacy personnel are pleased with his progress and relieved that the adversarial process is

---

Table 6.1

Positive Behavior Support Plan Parameters for Ray

General guidelines: Personal interactions (e.g., treat Ray warmly and with respect; provide assistance on tasks with which he has difficulty; give him choices, talk in short, clear sentences); communication (e.g., encourage use of words for requests, encourage use of multiple-word phrases and sentences); and social skills (e.g., stress courtesy and voice volume).

Decelerated (problem behaviors): The positive behavior support plan provides a table in which the following are described for each of the three problem behaviors (i.e., agitation, self-injurious behavior, and inappropriate attention getting): definition with examples, antecedents, hypothesized functions, prevention strategies, intervention strategies, and what to record on the accompanying data sheets.

Accelerated (replacement) behaviors: The positive behavior support plan also provides a table in which the following are described for each of the three accelerated behaviors (i.e., self-help skills, purposive behavior [at-home activities], and community activities: definition with examples, activities, procedures, necessary environmental adaptations, positive consequences, and what to record on the accompanying data sheets.

Data sheet: A one-page data sheet was developed on the basis of staff input that allows easy shift or hourly recording of each of the decelerated and accelerated behaviors.

---

over. The state Department of Developmental Disabilities is pleased and relieved as well, and the direct-care staff are much more optimistic and effective, because they have both helped developed and "bought into" the positive behavior support plan. As with other examples described in this book, clinical judgment not only is a key component of best practices, but it can also lead to win-win situations. Guidelines for this clinical judgment strategy are presented in Table 6.2.

Table 6.2
Guidelines Regarding Intervention Best Practices

1. Use a wholistic approach to the person.

2. Conduct the analyses with input from the person and significant others.

3. Integrate the results of the analyses into a clearly stated intervention strategy.

4. Familiarize all people involved with the key aspects of the strategy.

5. Evaluate person-referenced outcomes and use that information as "formative feedback" to all stakeholders for continuous improvement.

CHAPTER 7

Individualized Supports Planning, Implementation, and Evaluation: The Judge and Judy

Overview

Since the 1980s the supports paradigm has significantly influenced education and rehabilitation efforts in two ways: First, the level or intensity of a person's support needs has become the basis for decisions regarding the individualization of educational and rehabilitation efforts, including agency and systems planning and reimbursement patterns. Second, the supports orientation has brought together the related practices of person-centered planning, personal growth and development, community inclusion, and empowerment. This emphasis on supports and systems of supports is consistent with psychological and social models. Psychologically the concept of supports is in harmony with the "zone of proximal development," defined as the distance between the individual's independence and assisted problem-solving levels. As discussed by Scharnhorst and Buchel (1990), an individual's functioning can be increased significantly as a result of comparing the tasks the person can solve to the tasks the person could solve with the help of a more capable member of society. Socially the concept of supports is consistent with communitarianism, which tempers the excesses of individualism with an assertion of the rights of others in the larger society (Turnbull & Brunk, 1997).

The planning, implementing, and evaluating of individualized supports is occurring even as the field is experiencing a significant shift in thinking about individuals with mental retardation. This changed thinking is characterized by:

- a focus on person-centered planning, which emphasizes personal growth and development, choices, decisions, and empowerment;
- an ecological approach to disability that stresses the power of person-environmental interactions and the reduction of functional and activity limitations through person centered support strategies;
- a quality revolution that emphasizes personal well-being, quality of life, and valued outcomes; and
- the provision of services and supports in natural environments, based on the principles of inclusion and equity.

Supports "are resources and strategies that aim to promote the development, education, interests, and personal well-being of a person and that enhance individual functioning" (Luckasson et al., 2002, p. 15). The sources of support can include the person him- or herself, family and friends, colleagues, neighbors, and services. Services are one type of support provided by professionals and agencies; as we will see in Judy's case, the potential of natural supports is often overlooked.

The Case of Judy

Fortunately the district judge referenced in chapter 1 was willing to postpone his judgment on the parental rights of the single mother (Judy) until sufficient information could be collected for him to make his informed decision. During this time there was an opportunity to do nontraditional assessment and observation of Judy interacting with her child; complete a thorough social history that identified strengths, limitations, and potential sources of support; assess her profile and intensity of needed supports; and work with her maternal grandmother, who became a linchpin in the support systems eventually developed for Judy and her daughter. These activities led to sets of data and information that helped us understand Judy and her situation better. Among the more important:

- Judy graduated from her local high school's special education program. Earlier diagnoses varied and included learning disabled and educationally mentally handicapped and epilepsy (which has been well controlled since the age of 5). She currently lives in a supported living apartment provided jointly by the family and the state Department of Social Services.

- Her strengths include good social skills, strong motivation, good self-concept, good receptive language, her desire to be a mother, and a history of successful job performance across a number of part-time work experiences. Although working part time, Judy qualifies for public assistance.

- Limitations include limited expressive language, few friends, weaknesses in math and financial planning, and a short attention span. Additionally her family and neighbors were concerned about her epilepsy; "what would happen if she had a seizure?"

- Judy's child is by all indications normal and is in good health. After the birth Judy and the child bonded for several months; the child was then placed in foster care by the local welfare office.

- Although Judy's parents want nothing to do with the child (the notoriety of the pregnancy had been quite embarrassing), they are supportive of Judy in all other respects. Fortunately Judy's maternal grandmother and her grandmother's circle of friends were interested in Judy and the child and indicated during interviews their willingness to provide help to keep the two together.

As shown in the next section, the judgment part of this case included the recommendation that with appropriate individualized supports, Judy could be an adequate parent. The strategic part of competent clinical judgment required developing an individualized support plan (described later in the chapter) that would (a) meet Judy and the child's needs; (b) resolve the concerns expressed by Judy's parents, neighbors, the welfare agency; and (c) answer the judge's question: "What is your recommendation?"

The focus of the judge's question was on supports planning. Answering the question and developing the support plan involved critical thinking skills related to evaluation, interpretation, and explanation, and personal characteristics related to open-mindedness, analyticity, and inquisitiveness.

Clinical Judgment Actions

Clarify and State Precisely the Question(s) Set Before You

The judge's question was clear and stated precisely: "What is your recommendation regarding Judy being able to take care of the child?" Although it was basically a yes or no question, a key consideration was the precision, accuracy, and integrity of the recommendation and the individualized support plan.

Use a Relevant Framework for the Statement of the Question

Although a number of clinical judgment strategies—applying broad-based assessment strategies, conducting a thorough social history (including interviews with the grandmother and her friends), and reflecting cultural competence—were used to answer the judge's question, the principal strategy involved evaluating Judy's profile and intensity of support needs and then determining how they could be met given her current skills and environmentally based service and support networks. The evaluation was done within the context of the supports paradigm (as described earlier in this chapter) and included a profile of needed supports, an indication of the support functions that needed to be provided, and the identification of desired personal outcomes for Judy and the child. Once this was done, a recommendation could be made.

Conduct Needed Activities

It is helpful to think about a four-component process for assessing the pattern and intensity of needed supports. Using that information one can develop an individualized supports plan. These four components are as follows (Thompson et al., 2002):

- Identify desired life experiences and goals. In Judy's case, this was to be a successful mother and to have a full-time job.
- Determine the pattern and intensity of support needs. Support

areas will vary depending on both the person and his or her desired life experiences and goals. For Judy, critical areas included parenting, functional academics, memory aids, health maintenance, social involvement, and work. For others, the support areas might include exceptional medical or behavioral needs, home living, community living, life-long learning, employment, health and safety, social, and/or protection and advocacy. As part of this second component, it is also necessary to determine the intensity of the needed supports, which can be accomplished by determining the frequency, daily support time, and type of support required in each support area.

- Develop an individualized support plan. The data for such a plan comes from the second component along with input regarding potential providers of the supports. The analysis of these data (in next action step) will help determine the viability and potential of the proposed support plan; one can base a recommendation on that analysis.
- Monitor progress. A plan is only a plan until it is implemented and evaluated. Implementation is generally through a team process. Key factors to consider in the evaluation of the plan include the extent to which: (a) the desired life experiences and goals are being realized; (b) desired life experiences and goals remain relevant; and (c) the individualized support plan is implemented and changes made based on experiences with it.

In Judy's case, the primary areas of needed support were parenting, functional academics, memory aids, health maintenance, social involvement, and a job. Each of these six areas of support was assessed on three variables (Thompson et al., 2004): (a) Judy's currently expressed skills and limitations; (b) the frequency (none or < monthly; at least once a month but not once a week; at least once a week but not once a day; at least once a day but not once an hour; hourly or more frequently), duration or daily support time (none; < 30 min; 30 min to < 2 hr; 2 hr to < 4 hr; 4 hr or more), and type of support (none; monitoring; verbal/gestural prompting; partial physical assistance; full physical assistance); and (c) potential source of the support (i.e., the person responsible for providing the

73

support activity). Many of the needed supports can be provided by Judy through the strengths described earlier; however, some of the support activities that involve daily provision and daily or weekly monitoring would require support from someone else. Most activities could be provided in less than 2 hours per session.

Analyze the Data

Analyzing the data obtained from the supports assessment, it was apparent that although Judy needed considerable support to be both a successful mother and employee, such was possible given her support network. The extensiveness of this support network is shown in the individualized support plan summarized in Table 7.1. Due to the judge's concerns about Judy's limited attention span and verbal skills in relation to a small child, provision was made in the individualized support plan for overnight supervision if Judy and the grandmother thought this was necessary. Fortunately such supervision could be provided by staff from a nearby community residence for people with developmental disabilities. In addition, a med alert device was purchased and worn by Judy, along with a direct, color-coded telephone line to her grandmother and another friend.

Develop a Decision or Recommendation

Twelve sources of support were identified in the individualized support plan summarized in Table 7.1. The decision to recommend that Judy be granted parental rights and that she could take care of her child was based on a number of factors including the validity of the supports assessment, the extensiveness of Judy's support network, Judy's strengths and strong motivation to be a mother, and the commitment of members of the support network to "make it work for Judy." This information and data provided a strong basis for answering the judge's question and doing so with a high degree of certainty and precision. The judge was receptive to the recommendation, because it met the three criteria of good clinical judgment: that it be systematic, formal, and transparent.

Table 7.1 Judy's Individualized Support Plan			
Support Area	**Supports Provided**	**Frequency**	**Person Responsible for Monitoring**
Parenting	Well-baby clinic	Daily (M–F)	Judy and clinic
	Early intervention program (home training)	Daily (M–F)	Education services unit
	Baby-sitting services	During work	Grandmother and circle of friends
Functional academics	Speech therapy/ augmentative system	Weekly	Teacher volunteer
	Help with checkbook	Weekly	Case manager
Memory aids	Daily schedule Appointment book	Daily Weekly	Judy and grandmother Case manager
Health maintenance	Med-alert for seizure Smoke detectors	Daily Monthly	Judy and grandmother Neighbor
	Automated pill dispenser	Weekly	Judy and grandmother
	Emergency call service	Ongoing	Parents
Social activities	Community activities	Weekly	Local self-advocacy group, grandmother, parents, and friends
Job	Transportation	Daily (M–F)	Coworker

Communicate the Decision or Recommendation

Implementing the recommendation involved the following skills: (a) written communication to all stakeholders including the judge and all responsible individuals listed in Table 7.1; (b) negotiation, working with the family and the local Department of Social Welfare to convince them that with the support plan outlined in Table 7.1 Judy could be both a successful mother and employee; (c) preparation and presentation of Judy's individualized support plan to the judge; the presentation included leading the discussion as to its development, components, and chances of success; and (d) commitment to participate in the plan's implementation, monitoring, and evaluation. With this information, the judge granted Judy parental custody of the child with the provision that there be ongoing monitoring and evaluation and frequent reports submitted to the court. Thus both the judge's question and decision were made with increased certainty and precision.

Summary and Guidelines

Judy's case is not unique. As individuals with mental retardation have entered more directly into the mainstream of life, complex issues and questions regarding guardianship, parenting, voting, driving, and full-employment have emerged. These are issues that cannot be answered easily only on the basis of a psychometric test or clinical interview. Indeed, answering these questions and resolving the complex issues require something more: clinical judgment. In addition to strategies related to broad-based assessments, a thorough social history, best-practice intervention strategies, cultural competence, and aligning data and its collection to the critical questions asked, clinical judgment requires data related to the pattern and intensity of needed supports that will allow a person's identified desired life experiences and goals to become a reality.

Judy is now a successful single parent and a valued employee due in great part to the use of the fifth clinical judgment strategy:

planning, implementation, and evaluating individualized supports. Judy's case also reflects the fact that the application of clinical judgment involves a number of actions that result not only in good decision making, but also best practices. In furthering those best practices, the reader will find six support guidelines listed in Table 7.2.

Table 7.2
Support Guidelines

Supports should:

1. Be based on a thorough supports assessment in multiple life areas.

2. Be individualized and reflect the pattern and intensity of needed supports across multiple life areas.

3. Be sensitive to culturally based behaviors and beliefs.

4. Blend natural and service-based supports.

5. Focus on outcomes related to independence, relationships, contributions, school and community participation, and personal well-being.

6. Integrate personal, technical, environmental, and behaviorally based sources of support.

CHAPTER 8

Cultural Competence and Linguistic Diversity: Does Ezra Have Mental Retardation or Developmental Delay?

Overview

Our citizenry is becoming more diverse, and with that diversity comes a plethora of values, behaviors, and traditions. Although diversity is increasingly valued in most communities, language and cultural diversity can present a real challenge to the clinician. For example, most of our current standardized instruments for measuring intelligence and adaptive behavior generally do not reflect cultural or linguistic diversity, including the norms used for comparative purposes. In addition, there is frequently a mismatch between the clinician's language and culture and that of the person being evaluated, resulting in a lack of sensitivity to—or awareness of—subtle cultural or linguistic nuances. Thus, for people like Ezra, the clinician needs to consider how her assessment can use appropriate instruments that are sensitive to the language and culture of the person, be proficient in the individual's language and culture, involve the use of a trained interpreter if necessary, and be conducted at a location comfortable for the family.

A consensus is emerging about how clinicians can respond competently to the challenges presented by cultural and linguistic diversity. Important components of this consensus found in the published literature (e.g., Baca & Cervantes, 2004; Ibrahim, 1995;

Kleinhert & Farmer-Kearns, 2001; Luckasson et al., 2002; Lynch & Hanson, 1992; Salvia & Ysseldyke, 2004; Schuman, 2002; Sirotnik, 2002; Tassé & Craig, 1999) are the following:

- In making a valid assessment, consider the individual's culture, ethnicity, and customs.
- Ensure the participation of necessary cultural informants or consultants, and make necessary language accommodations in regard to the assessments.
- Use multiple sources of information about the individual, including customs that might influence assessment results.
- Understand the transactions between parents and program personnel around defining the person's status, considering their preferences, expectations, and demands particular to each setting.
- Be sensitive to the distortions of the current approach for individuals based on "mainstream values" and the impasse in communication brought about by the conflict in cultural constructions of human growth and development.
- Be aware of one's own cultural orientation, focus, and bias while appreciating and respecting cultural differences; interact and communicate in a sensitive fashion.
- View intercultural experiences as learning opportunities as one helps to develop an individualized assessment plan that respects culture and language.

Despite this emerging consensus, a significant danger remains. It is still too easy to overlook genuine disability by permitting language and culture to overshadow it (Collier, 1998; Luckasson et al., 2002). Thus a clinician needs to reflect on his or her own culture and language and the ways they affect him or her and be vigilant against superficial conclusions that limit an accurate assessment of the person's disability. In that regard, the clinician must avoid the potential for "cultural or linguistic overshadowing" to operate and thus be a detriment to the individual's welfare. For example, a person whose disability is overlooked by cultural or linguistic overshadowing will unfairly be excluded from essential services, protections, and benefits to which he or she is entitled. As we discussed in chapter 1 in reference to the contraindications of clinical judgment, "clinical judgment" should not be used as a justification for abbreviated evaluations, a vehicle for stereotypes or prejudices, a substitute for insufficiently explored questions, an excuse for incomplete or missing data, or a way to solve political problems.

The Case of Ezra

Ezra and his family live on Native American lands in a geographically isolated area of a western state. Ezra was born several weeks early, in the family vehicle stopped on the side of a rural road. His mother had gone into labor at the family ranch. The entire family had immediately embarked on the four-hour trip to the distant hospital but was unable to make it in time. Ezra and his mother arrived at the hospital two hours after his birth and received necessary care. The pediatrician noted nearly normal developmental signs in Ezra, and he and his mother went home 36 hours later.

Ezra is now 4 years old, and his family has become increasingly concerned about his abilities. He is not able to effectively accomplish ordinary chores at the family home. For example, he forgets to feed the dog; he leaves the horse corral gate open; he uses the last of the water without telling anyone; he cannot write his name. The worried family brought him to the elementary school 45 miles from its ranch and asked that he be allowed to begin school early in order to fix these problems. The school can admit him only if he qualifies as eligible for early intervention services in a specific category, such as mental retardation or a developmental delay. The school outreach worker minimizes Ezra's apparent deficits, attributing the limitations to his culture. But the school psychologist is concerned and has proposed a multidisciplinary team meeting with the family to design an in-depth culturally sensitive assessment.

Does Ezra have mental retardation or a developmental delay, making him eligible for early intervention services? Because Ezra is from a Native American family that has taught Ezra only his native language, and because the school's majority population, as well as the school psychologist, is Anglo, attempting to answer this question requires the clinician to use clinical judgment. The focus of the question is diagnosis. Throughout the team's activities, the critical thinking skills needed include analysis, evaluation, inference, interpretation, and explanation. The intended products are team input and a written report regarding the diagnosis and suggested formulation of an individualized support plan for Ezra.

Clinical Judgment Actions

Clarify and State Precisely the Question Set Before You

The questions asked in Ezra's case are very straightforward. Does Ezra have mental retardation or developmental delay, and does he meet the eligibility criteria for early intervention services?

Use a Relevant Framework for the Statement of the Question

When an individual's language or culture is diverse, the evaluation team must take particular care to ensure that any assessment plan addresses the individual's abilities or disabilities, not simply the culture or language. This means that the team must create a plan that will: collect relevant information about the person and the home environment and/or language; analyze the demands of the proposed environment and language; complete a thorough social history that includes culture and language; select suitable test instruments and outline necessary assessment modifications or accommodations; provide an evaluator(s) sensitive to the person's language and culture; and ensure that the assessment plan is implemented in a manner consistent with all legal and ethical guidelines.

For preschool and school-aged children who are assessed for special education services, the most relevant law is the Individuals With Disabilities Education Act (IDEA; 2004). IDEA is clear on requirements for nonbiased assessment. "Materials and procedures used to assess a child with limited English proficiency [must be] selected and administered to ensure that they measure the extent to which the child has a disability and needs special education, rather than measuring the child's English language skills" (§ 300.532(a)(2)). The law requires that to the extent feasible the tests must be administered in the child's first language or mode of communication. Limited proficiency in English alone is specifically prohibited as a justification for provision of special education services.

For adults, the legal principles are the same, but they are not necessarily embodied in a particular statute. Federal nondiscrimination legislation, such as § 504 of the Rehabilitation Act (1973) and the Americans With Disabilities Act (1990) may be relevant, and state human rights legislation may also be applicable.

Typically, as in the case of Ezra, the question being asked focuses on the person's disabilities or current academic achievement. Sometimes, however, the question focuses on culture. Culture is the total combination of influences, such as ethnicity, gender, religion, and economic background (Payne, 1996), in which the person has developed. Because culture can affect an individual's behaviors and beliefs, an understanding of culture is essential to interpreting actions and understanding. Even for those who appear to be "acculturated," people can range in the degree of acculturation from significantly less acculturated to highly acculturated (Collier, 1998). Individuals can show acculturation by being: (a) bicultural (holding two cultures without deterioration of either), (b) assimilated (rejecting original culture and accepting new culture), (c) traditional (rejecting new culture and holding original culture), and (d) marginal (rejecting both new and original culture).

Other times, however, the question is about language proficiency. The questions may be how proficient is the person in English and, in which language the assessment is best conducted. It is critical to consider different levels of English language proficiency, even when the person appears to be comfortable in English. According to Cummins (1999), an individual may have only basic interpersonal communication skills (BICS), which require 2 to 3 years to acquire. The more advanced cognitive academic language proficiency (CALP) requires 5 to 7 years to acquire. Other times, the question might be how proficient an individual is in his home language. Assessments to determine language proficiency raise significant issues but are beyond the scope of this volume.

Conduct Needed Activities

Due to the conditions surrounding Ezra's birth and his current behavior, the initial hypothesis tested was that Ezra was a child with developmental delay. To test this hypothesis, a bilingual pediatrician who speaks Ezra's home language was asked to do a developmental exam focusing on key developmental milestones including gross and fine motor skills, ambulation, sensory functioning, nutrition, and growth patterns. Based on this evaluation, the pediatrician concluded that a diagnosis of developmental delay, while supported, did not sufficiently account for Ezra's problems, and became more concerned about Ezra's apparent deficits in adaptive behavior and intelligence.

According to the 2002 American Association on Mental Retardation system, "Mental retardation is a disability characterized by significant limitations both in intellectual functioning and in adaptive behavior as expressed in conceptual, social, and practical adaptive skills. This disability originates before age 18" (Luckasson et al., p. 1). To assess Ezra's adaptive behavior, the team selected the Vineland Adaptive Behavior Scale—Form S (VABS–S; Sparrow, Balla, & Cicchetti, 1984). Form S was deemed appropriate for a number of reasons including: (a) its conversational data-gathering format, used as the basis for interviewing Ezra's parents; (b) its available norms that reflect age, gender, ethnicity, parental education, geographical region, and community size; and (c) psychometric data (reliability and validity) that are very good for Form S. The team concluded that the assessment of Ezra's adaptive behavior was culture- and language-fair, because it used an interview format with the parents and because Ezra's adaptive behavior profile was compared to community norms. On the VABS–S, Ezra demonstrated significant limitations on adaptive behavior.

In regard to intelligence, Ezra's cultural and language diversity required the use of an assessment instrument that does not depend heavily on verbal language for the examiner or examinee. For that reason, the Leiter International Performance Scale—Revised (Leiter–

R; Reid & Miller, 1997) was employed. This instrument is reported to measure fluid intelligence, which is thought to be less influenced by education, social background, or family experiences. The Leiter–R is designed to be used with individuals aged 2 to 21 and has good internal consistency, reliability, and concurrent validity. On the visualization and reasoning battery of the Leiter–R, Ezra's estimated IQ was shown to be significantly impaired. Attention and memory domains were not administered due to their reliance on language, comprehension, and verbal expression.

Analyze the Data

One of the initial issues is whether the individual's performance is a result of diversity. Certainly that possibility must be considered. But it is equally important that the person not be denied valuable benefits or services if he does have a disability (because of an unsubstantiated claim that the assessment results are a reflection of culture or language).

Analyzing the data can be particularly challenging when modifications or accommodations have been made because of the person's language or culture. Despite these challenges, Ezra's significant limitations in both adaptive behavior and intelligence suggest strongly the diagnosis of mental retardation; he is eligible for services, and because of the early age and the tentativeness of his diagnosis, continued refinement of assessment is indicated.

Develop a Decision or Recommendation

Any recommendation must be supported by documentation of an assessment that has addressed any diversity issues. Ezra is clearly eligible for early intervention services, but the precise diagnosis remains tentative because of his early age. The importance of differentiation between a diagnosis of mental retardation and developmental delay varies from state to state. In some states either diagnosis may result in the same service eligibility. Even so, thorough diagnostic assessment and good clinical judgment can benefit the child and family. As for the family, more precision in a diagnosis will assist parental understanding of Ezra's condition, planning for the future, supporting the health of the family and future children, and stress management. As for the child, a clear understanding of Ezra's condition can eventually make a big difference in laying the groundwork for understanding the cause of the disability, supporting his transitional processes, and perhaps improving a match to successful interventions.

Communicate the Decision or Recommendation

Ezra's teacher must remember that diagnoses at such an early age are imprecise, and the focus should be on his learning and success in school and at home. Subsequent reevaluations are essential. This work will set the stage for a more assured diagnosis by age 9, when a precise disability area will be required for special school services. The teacher must juggle several issues such as Ezra's current learning needs and the necessity to continue diagnostic precision. Now that eligibility is established, a supports plan must be implemented as described in chapter 7.

Summary and Guidelines

The primary purpose of diagnosis is to develop an intervention plan that will benefit the individual and lead to needed supports. Supports providers should think beyond the diagnosis and pursue enhanced functioning. A major diagnostic concern is that the individual's disabilities will be overlooked, because the person's challenges are attributed to his diversity rather than to his disability. The intent of this chapter has been to emphasize that good clinical practice, including good clinical judgment, must be employed to prevent that from happening. As discussed throughout the chapter, it is important to consider all aspects of the broad-based assessment, develop differential hypotheses, and continue to test, confirm, or reject the hypotheses. As reflected in the guidelines summarized in Table 8.1, cultural competence and linguistic diversity are key elements of clinical judgment.

Table 8.1
Cultural Competence and Linguistic Diversity Guidelines

1. Know and follow all legal and regulatory requirements for nonbiased assessment.

2. Know and follow the ethical requirements and standards of your profession concerning diversity and assessment.

3. Be familiar with the strengths and limitations of a broad range of tests and assessment strategies for individuals of diverse cultural and linguistic backgrounds.

4. Use assessment instruments that are sensitive to diversity, have norms that are based on diverse groups, and have acceptable psychometric properties.

5. Investigate and understand the culture, the degree of acculturation, and the language of the individual, and the ways they affect the person.

6. Do not allow cultural or linguistic diversity to overshadow or minimize actual disability.

PART 3
Putting It All Together

We anticipate this book being used by numerous groups in various ways. We foresee, for example, its use by clinicians who as part of a professional team want to ensure best practices in diagnosis, classification, and the planning of individualized supports. We can also see it being used by educators and school psychologists to guide special education assessments and decisions resulting from those assessments. Third, we see it being used as a framework in forensic evaluations, as clinicians grapple with the complexities involved in legal definitions and determinations. Fourth, we anticipate its use by professors who want their students to demonstrate the clinical judgment strategies and actions outlined in the preceding six chapters. Challenges commonly faced by these user groups are those we addressed throughout the text: formal assessment that is less than optimal; complex medical or behavioral conditions that require multiple analyses; legal restrictions that significantly impact opportunities to assess the person within the context of community environments typical of the individual's age peers and culture; and cultural and/or linguistic differences that limit the obtaining of valid assessment information.

CHAPTER 9

Facilitating the Clinical Judgment Process

Key Points About Clinical Judgment

Throughout the book we have stressed that the use of clinical judgment is one of the four competencies involved in best practices. The other three are (a) incorporating professional standards, (b) aligning with professional ethics, and (c) basing one's actions on research-based knowledge. As shown in Figure 1.1, clinical judgment plays a variable role in best practices, and the amount of emphasis on clinical judgment will vary depending on the (a) amount of information, (b) type of information, (c) complexity of the issue, and (d) qualifications, experience, and expertise of the clinician. We have also emphasized that clinical judgment is a special type of judgment rooted in a high level of clinical expertise and experience, and that it emerges directly from extensive data. As reflected in the cases on which the preceding six chapters were based, clinical judgment is acquired through the clinician's explicit training, direct experience with person(s) with whom the clinician is working, and familiarity with the person's life and environment.

We have also cautioned throughout the text that clinical judgment should not be thought of as a justification for abbreviated evaluations, a vehicle for stereotypes or prejudices, a substitute for insufficiently explored questions, an excuse for incomplete or missing data, or a way to solve political problems. Rather, clinical judgment is characterized by its being systematic (i.e., organized, sequential, and logical), formal (i.e., explicit and reasoned), and transparent (i.e., apparent and communicated clearly). Thus clinical judgment is an essential component of best practices and a process that enhances the accuracy of decision making in complex situations involving diagnosis, classification, supports provision, and research-based evidence.

Incorporating Clinical Judgment Into Best Practices

If the overall purpose of clinical judgment is to ensure best practices by enhancing the precision, accuracy, and integrity of the clinician's decision in a particular case, how might the multiple users of this book facilitate that process? We suggest that whether the process is centered on the acquisition, demonstration, or evaluation of clinical judgment, the particular user needs to focus clearly on the strategies, actions, and guidelines discussed throughout the text and summarized as follows. Note that for each strategy, action, and corresponding clinical judgment guidelines, the user is asked to answer one or more critical questions related to the incorporation of clinical judgment into best practices.

Clinical Judgment Strategies

Whether one focuses on the acquisition, demonstration and use, or evaluation of the six clinical judgment strategies presented in the text, several key questions relate to each.

1. **Conducting a thorough social history.** Did the social history address all aspects of the issues related to the individual's functioning? Did it take a wholistic approach to understanding the person's life, family, environments, and circumstances?

2. **Aligning data and its collection to the question at hand.** For diagnosis-related questions, does the information pertain to intelligence and adaptive functioning and age of onset? For classification-related questions, does the information pertain to competency indicators, support indicators, intelligence subdomains, adaptive behavior profiles, and/or etiology-risk

factors? For supports-related questions, does the information pertain to profiles of needed supports, the intensity of those needed supports, and personal and valued outcomes related to the provision of supports? Additionally, did the measures used have acceptable psychometric properties?

3. **Applying broad-based assessment strategies.** Were an appropriate wide range of behavioral observation, assessment, and recording strategies used to evaluate the person? Were standards used that involve broad outcomes related to real-life application and that can be applied across age and environmental situations? Was assessment linked to intervention, and was the individual involved directly in the assessment process?

4. **Implementing intervention best practices.** Is the proposed intervention(s) formulated on research-based knowledge, the modern vision of individuals with mental retardation as complex human beings with strengths and limitations, and an ecological (person-environment) perspective? Is the proposed intervention based on descriptive, functional, ecological, and outcomes analyses?

5. **Planning, implementing, and evaluating individualized supports.** Is there a clear description of the evaluation procedure used to determine the pattern and intensity of needed supports? Does the individualized support plan cover the major life activity areas, involve multiple support functions, and include personal outcomes?

6. **Reflecting cultural competence and linguistic diversity.** Does the assessment plan address the individual's strengths and limitations and not simply the culture or language? In addition, does the assessment plan: (a) collect relevant information about the person and his home environment and language, (b) select suitable test instruments and outline necessary assessment modifications and accommodations, and (c) provide an evaluator who is sensitive to the person's language and culture?

Clinical Judgment Operational Actions

Implementing each of these six clinical judgment strategies involves the use of the six operational actions discussed throughout the text. Basic to their use is (a) a clear understanding of the question asked (i.e., is its focus diagnosis, classification, or supports planning?); (b) the judicious use of critical thinking skills related to analysis, evaluation, inference, interpretation, and explanation; and (c) an understanding of the intended or anticipated product (e.g., verbal report, written report, or team input). In the acquisition, demonstration and use, and evaluation of these actions, the following key questions about each should be kept in mind and answered.

1. **Clarify and state precisely the question set before you.** Clinicians may need to use a variety of strategies to clarify questions. Strategies might include asking for the question in writing, requesting further explanation, researching the specifics of the question, agreeing on the definition of particular terms, restating the question and confirming the restatement, consulting with others who understand the question better, and testing one's understanding in other ways. The key question is "Is there a clear mutual understanding of all aspects of the inquiry?"

2. **Use a relevant framework for the statement of the question(s).** Questions asked of clinicians cannot be answered in isolation; one needs to understand a question's context and framework. Typically this contextual framework may be derived from legal requirements, research-theoretical constructs, statements from authoritative organizations, or statements of public policy. The key two-part question is "Can one identify the framework in which the question is rooted?" and "Is the framework for the answer explicitly aligned with the framework for the question?" At that point, one can identify the needed activities.

3. **Conduct needed activities.** When clinicians design a plan and conduct the needed activities, they must ensure that each exercise is consistent with the three characteristics of clinical judgment: (a) systematic (i.e., organized, sequential, and

logical); (b) formal (i.e., explicit and reasoned); and (c) transparent (i.e., apparent and communicated clearly). Thus, for this action, the key question is "Did the activities conducted meet these three clinical judgment criteria?" If so, one's data reflect certainty and precision.

4. **Analyze data.** The analysis of the data used by the clinician in reaching his or her decision or recommendation should reflect the same characteristics as just listed in reference to conducting the needed activities: systematic, formal, and transparent. In addition, proper data analysis requires: (a) use of the scientific method and its emphasis on empiricism and hypothesis testing and (b) critical thinking skills related to inference and interpretation. The key question for this action is "Were the three criteria of systematic, formal, and transparent met, and did the analysis and its interpretation involve the scientific method and critical thinking skills?" If so, one has a valid basis for a decision or recommendation.

5. **Develop a decision or recommendation.** A clinician's decision or recommendation can involve a number of purposes including answering those questions related to diagnosis, classification, and supports planning (Luckasson et al., 2002). For diagnosis, common purposes include establishing eligibility for services, benefits, and/or legal protections. For classification, common purposes include grouping individuals for service reimbursement or funding, research, services, and/or communication about selected characteristics. For planning supports, the most common purpose is to enhance personal outcomes related to independence, relationships, contributions, school and community participation, and personal well-being. The key question regarding this fifth action is whether the decision or recommendation: (a) is clearly focused on diagnosis, classification, and/or planning supports and (b) answers the question asked.

6. **Communicate the decision or recommendation.** Our experiences over the years suggest three important aspects of

communicating one's decision or recommendation. The key question for this action is "Does one's decision and recommendation meet these three criteria?" If so, the decision or recommendation can be communicated with increased certainty and precision (and credibility). The criteria are as follows:

- First, have integrity. Do not promise more than you can deliver; point out the equivocal nature of the data (if such is the case) and attempt to explain why.

- Second, be competent. Use those strategies, actions, and guidelines that reflect this clinical judgment component of best practice.

- Third, consider the requirements related to a clear focus of the question, the critical thinking skills required to establish the framework for answering the question, and the form of the intended product.

Clinical Judgment Guidelines

Competent clinical judgment needs to be anchored within a broad set of clinical judgment guidelines that are based not only on research-based knowledge, professional codes of ethics, and professional standards, but also on the clinical judgment strategies and actions just summarized. The purpose of these guidelines is to provide clinicians with a guide and standard that will facilitate good decision making based on the clinician's training and expertise, the assessment data obtained, and the clinician's experiences with the person. The guidelines can also be considered as a benchmark against which to evaluate clinical judgment practices to ensure that they are truly consistent with best practices. Important guidelines were presented in tabular form at the end of each of the preceding six chapters. For the reader's convenience, they are listed in total in the appendix. The critical question that multiple users should ask about these guidelines is "How can they be used in the clinical work that I do or in the evaluation of clinical judgment used by others?"

Conclusion

We hope the reader has gained an appreciation for both clinical judgment and the need for a book on this topic for the field of mental retardation. Such a book is critical today due to a number of trends impacting the field, including: (a) the power struggle and shifting alliances between self-advocates and professionals, (b) the competing models of disability, (c) the conflicting values expressed by participants involved in the inclusion and empowerment movement, (d) questions about the modern application of traditional scientific approaches, (e) conflicting models of resource allocation, and (f) challenges to the future of traditional professions. We hope also that this text has addressed those issues, presented the rationale and components of clinical judgment, and explored why there is a need to explicate clinical judgment at this time.

Clinical judgment is part of a dynamic diagnostic and problem-solving process. In this book we have attempted to describe a set of strategies, actions, and guidelines that clinicians can use across different situations as a basis for answering challenging questions, developing difficult decisions and recommendations, and demonstrating best practices. We trust that using these strategies, actions, and guidelines will lead to more transparent analyses and increasingly logical and principled decisions and recommendations.

APPENDIX

Clinical Judgment Guidelines

Conduct a thorough social history.

1. Clarify any legal question and the form the recommendations should take.

2. Be aware of current legal findings and definitions.

3. Investigate, collect, and organize all relevant informaton about the person's life including stages, trajectory, development, functioning, relationships, and family.

4. Explore the possible reasons for differences in data, including (a) poorly trained examiner, (b) improper generalization of test scores administered for other purposes, (c) improper selection of tests, (d) neglect of consideration of standard error of measurement, (e) mistakes in scoring, (f) administrations of the same test too close in time, (g) different editions of the same test and resultant Flynn effects, (h) bias, and (i) behavioral differences in the individual.

5. Develop contemporary assessment, if indicated, in order to show changes in functioning over the life span.

Align data and its collection to the critical questions asked.

1. Understand clearly what question is being asked and what data will be required to answer it.

2. Establish one's competence to pursue the clinical judgment actions that are required.

3. Use research-based knowledge to incorporate currently

available measures and strategies or use professional standards to develop needed data-collection techniques.

4. Use multiple data sources (e.g., personal appraisal or functional assessment) to obtain the necessary data.

5. Show clearly that the obtained data is aligned with the critical question(s) asked.

Apply broad-based assessment strategies.

1. Incorporate a broad evaluative strategy.

2. Use standards with broad outcomes that relate to real-life application and can be applied across age and situations; be flexible enough that you look at the real-life application respecting the person and demands.

3. Link assessment to instruction or intervention.

4. Involve the individual in self-assessment on a regular basis.

5. Assessments may be refined as the person's condition, status, or functioning changes.

Implement intervention best practices.

1. Use a wholistic approach to the person.

2. Conduct the analyses with input from the person and significant others.

3. Integrate the results of the analyses into a clearly stated intervention strategy.

4. Familiarize all people involved with the key aspects of the strategy.

5. Evaluate person-referenced outcomes and use that information as "formative feedback" to all stakeholders for continuous improvement.

Plan, implement, and evaluate individualized supports.

Supports should:

1. Be based on a thorough supports assessment in multiple life areas.
2. Be individualized and reflect the pattern and intensity of needed supports across multiple life areas.
3. Be sensitive to culturally based behaviors and beliefs.
4. Blend natural and service-based supports.
5. Focus on outcomes related to independence, relationships, contributions, school and community participation, and personal well-being.
6. Integrate personal, technical, environmental, and behaviorally based sources of support.

Reflect cultural competence and linguistic diversity.

1. Know and follow all legal and regulatory requirements for nonbiased assessment.
2. Know and follow the ethical requirements and standards of your profession concerning diversity and assessment.
3. Be familiar with the strengths and limitations of a broad range of tests and assessment strategies for individuals of diverse cultural and linguistic backgrounds.
4. Use assessment instruments that are sensitive to diversity, have norms that are based on diverse groups, and have acceptable psychometric properties.
5. Investigate and understand the culture, the degree of acculturation, and the language of the individual, and the ways they affect the person.
6. Do not allow cultural or linguistic diversity to overshadow or minimize actual disability.

References

Adoption Assistance and Child Welfare Act of 1980, Pub. L. No. 96-272. 42 U.S.C. § 620 *et seq.*, §§ 629, 670 *et seq.*, and §§ 136a and 136d.

American Geriatrics Society. (2001). Guidelines and position statements. In *The American Geriatrics Society, position statements.* Retrieved from http://www.americangeriatrics.org/products/positionpapers/index.shtml

American Medical Association. (2001). *Principles of medical ethics.* Washington, DC: American Medical Association House of Delegates.

American Nurses Association. (2001). *Code of ethics for nurses with interpretive statements.* Washington, DC: Author.

American Philosophical Association. (1990). Critical thinking: A statement of expert consensus for purposes of educational assessment and instruction. (ERIC Document Reproduction Service No. ED315423)

American Psychological Association. (1992). *Ethics code.* Washington, DC: Author.

American Psychological Association. (2002). Ethical principles of psychologists and code of conduct. *American Psychologist, 57,* 1060–1073.

American Speech-Language-Hearing Association. (2003). Code of ethics (Revised). *ASHA Supplement, 23,* 13–15.

Americans With Disabilities Act of 1990, 42 U.S.C.A. § 1210 *et seq.* (West 1993).

Assistive Technology Act of 1998, 29 U.S.C. § 1301 *et seq.*

Atkins v. Virginia, 536 U.S. 304 (2002).

Baca, L. M., & Cervantes, H. T. (2004). *The bilingual special education interface* (4th ed.). Upper Saddle River, NJ: Pearson Prentice Hall.

Benjamin, M., & Curtis, J. (1992). *Ethics in nursing* (3rd ed.). New York: Oxford University Press.

Brown v. Board of Education, 347 U.S. 483 (1954).

Children's and Communities Mental Health Systems Improvement Act, 42 U.S.C. § 290 *et seq.* (1994).

Collier, C. (1998). *Separating difference from disability: Assessing diverse learners.* Ferndale, WA: Cross-Cultural Developmental Education Services.

Cummins, J. (1999). *BICS and CALP: Clarifying the distinction.* (ERIC Document Reproduction Service No. ED438551)

Developmental Disabilities Assistance and Bill of Rights Act of 2000, 42 U.S.C. § 15001 *et seq.*

Facione, N. C., & Facione, P. A. (1996). Externalizing the critical thinking in clinical judgment. *Nursing Outlook, 44,* 129–136.

Goals 2000: Educate America Act of 1994, Pub. L. No. 103-227. 20 U.S.C. § 5801 *et seq.*

Henderson, C. M. (2004). Genetically linked syndromes in intellectual disabilities. *Journal of Policy and Practice in Intellectual Disabilities, 1*(1), 31–41.

Herr, S. S., O'Sullivan, J., & Hogan, C. (2002). A friend in court: The Association's role and judicial trends. In R. L. Schalock, P. C. Baker, & M. D. Croser (Eds.), *Embarking on a new century: Mental retardation at the end of the 20th century* (pp. 27–44). Washington, DC: American Association on Mental Retardation.

Home Care for Certain Disabled Children (Katie Beckett) Waivers, 42 U.S.C. § 1381 *et seq.* (1994).

Howe, K. R., & Miramontes, O. B. (1992). *The ethics of special education*. New York: Columbia University, Teachers College.

Ibrahim, E. A. (1995). Multicultural influences on rehabilitation training and services: The shift to valuing nondominant cultures. In O. C. Karan & S. Greenspan (Eds.), *Community rehabilitation services for people with disabilities* (pp. 145–168). Boston: Butterworth.

Improving America's Schools Act of 1994, Pub. L. No 103-382. 20 U.S.C. § 6301 *et seq.*

Individuals With Disabilities Education Act, 20 U.S.C. § 1400 *et seq.* (2004).

Jacobson, J. W., & Mulick, J. A. (1996). *Manual of diagnosis and professional practice in mental retardation*. Washington, DC: American Psychological Association.

Kleinhert, H. L., & Farmer-Kearns, J. (2001). *Alternate assessment: Measuring outcome and supports for students with disabilities*. Baltimore: Paul H. Brookes.

Luckasson, R., Borthwick-Duffy, S., Buntinx, W. H. E., Coulter, D. A., Craig, E. M., Reeve, A., Schalock, R. L., Snell, M. E., Spitalnik, D. M., Spreat, S., & Tassé, M. J. (2002). *Mental retardation: Diagnosis, classification, and systems of supports* (10th ed.). Washington, DC: American Association on Mental Retardation.

Luckasson, R., Coulter, D. A., Polloway, E. A., Reiss, S., Schalock, R. L., Snell, M. E., Spitalnik, D. M., & Stark, J. A. (1992). *Mental retardation: Diagnosis, classification, and systems of supports* (9th ed.). Washington, DC: American Association on Mental Retardation.

Lynch, E. W., & Hanson, M. J. (1992). *Developing cross-cultural competence: A guide for working with young children and their families*. Baltimore: Paul H. Brookes.

McIntyre, T., & Forness, S. R. (1996). Is there a new definition yet or are our kids still seriously emotionally disturbed? *Beyond Behavior, 7*(3), 4–9.

Menand, L. (2001). *The metaphysical club: A story of ideas in America.* New York: Farrar, Straus and Giroux.

National Association of Social Workers. (1996). *Code of ethics* (Rev. 1999). Washington, DC: Author.

National Board of Certified Counselors. (1997). *Code of ethics.* Washington, DC: Author.

National Career Development Association. (2003). *Consumer guidelines to selecting a career counselor.* Tulsa, OK: Creative Management Alliance. Retrieved from http://www.ncda.org/

National Education Association. (1975). *Code of ethics of the education profession.* Washington, DC: National Education Association 1975 Representative Assembly.

Newman, D. W., Kellett, S., & Beail, N. (2003). From research and development to practice-based evidence: Clinical governance initiatives in a service for adults with mild intellectual disability and mental health needs. *Journal of Intellectual Disability Research, 47*(1), 68–74.

Norris, S., & Ennis, R. (1989). *Evaluating critical thinking.* Pacific Grove, CA: Midwest Publications.

Olmstead v. L. C. 527 U.S. 581 (1999).

Omnibus Budget Reconciliation Act of 1987, Pub. L. No. 100-203.

Payne, R. (1996). *A framework for understanding poverty.* Highlands, TX: Process.

Rehabilitation Act of 1973, 29 U.S.C. § 794.

Reid, G. H., & Miller, L. J. (1997). *Leiter International Performance Scale–Revised.* Wood Dale, IL: Stoelting.

Reinders, J. S. (2002). The ethics of behaviour modification.

Journal of Intellectual Disability Research, 46(2), 187–190.

Salvia, J., & Ysseldyke, J. E. (2004). *Assessment in special and inclusive education* (9th ed.). Boston: Houghton Mifflin.

Schalock, R. L. (2001). Outcome-based evaluation (2nd ed.). New York: Kluwer-Plenum.

Schalock, R. L. (2004). The emerging disability paradigm and its implications for the policy and practice. *Journal of Disability Policy Studies, 14*(4), 204–215.

Schalock, R. L., Baker, P. C., & Croser, M. D. (2002). *Embarking on a new century: Mental retardation at the end of the 20th century.* Washington, DC: American Association on Mental Retardation.

Schalock, R. L., & Verdugo, M. A. (2002). *Handbook on quality of life for human service practitioners.* Washington, DC: American Association on Mental Retardation.

Scharnhorst, U., & Buchel, F. P. (1990). Cognitive and metacognitive components of learning: Search for the locus of retarded performance. *European Journal of Psychology of Education, 5,* 207–230.

Schuman, A. (2002). Help or hindrance? Staff perspectives on developmental assessment in multicultural early childhood settings. *Mental Retardation, 40*(4), 313–320.

Sirotnik, K. A. (2002, May). Promoting responsible accountability in schools and education. *Phi Delta Kappan,* 662–670.

Sparrow, S. S., Balla, D. A., & Cicchetti, D. V. (1984). *Vineland Adaptive Behavior Scales.* Circle Pines, MN: American Guidance Services.

Tassé, M. J., & Craig, E. M. (1999). Critical issues in the cross-cultural assessment of adaptive behavior. In R. L. Schalock (Ed.), *Adaptive behavior and its measurement: Implications for the field of mental retardation* (pp. 161–183). Washington, DC: American Association on Mental Retardation.

Thompson, J. R., Bryant, B. R., Campbell, E. M., Craig, E. M. et al. (2004). *Support Intensity Scale Assessment Manual.* Washington, DC: American Association on Mental Retardation.

Thompson, J. R., Hughes, C., Schalock, R. L., Silverman, W., Tassé, M. J., Bryant, B., Craig, E. M., & Campbell, E. M. (2002). Integrating supports in assessment and planning. *Mental Retardation, 40*(5), 390–405.

Ticket to Work and Work Incentives Improvement Act of 1999, Pub. L. No. 106-170. 42 U.S.C. §§ 1320b-19, 1396 *et seq.*

Title XIX (HCBS Waivers; Pub. L. No. 92-223) of the Social Security Act of 1971, 42 U.S.C. § 1396n(b).

Turnbull, H. R. III, & Brunk, G. L. (1997). Quality of life and public policy. In R. L. Schalock (Ed.), *Quality of life. Vol. 2: Application to persons with disabilities* (pp. 201–210). Washington, DC: American Association on Mental Retardation.

Turnbull, H. R. III, Wilcox, B. L., Stowe, M. J., & Umbarger, G. T. III. (2001). Matrix of federal statutes and federal and state court decisions reflecting the core concepts of disability policy. *Journal of Disability Policy Studies, 12*(3), 144–176.

Tymchuk, A. J., Lakin, K. C., & Luckasson, R. (2001). *The forgotten generation: The status and challenges of adults with mild cognitive limitations.* Baltimore: Paul H. Brookes.

Vehmas, S. (2004). Ethical analysis of the concept of disability. *Mental Retardation, 42*(3), 209–222.

Warren, S. F. (2002). Presidential address 2002—Genes, brains, and behavior: The road ahead. *Mental Retardation, 40*(6), 471–476.

Williams, J. M., & Murphy, P. (2000). Quality of life: A comprehensive model for rehabilitation assessment in litigation. *Journal of Forensic Vocational Analysis, 3*(1), 31–46.

Workforce Investment Partnership Act of 1998, 29 U.S.C. § 2801 *et seq.*

World Health Organization. (2001). *International classification of functioning, disability, and health* (ICF). Geneva: Author.

Wyatt v. Stickney (1972). 344 Supp. 373, 387 (M.D. Ala. 1972), *aff'd sub nom,* Wyatt v. Aderholt, 503 F.2d. 1305 (5th Cir.).

Subject Index

Assessment
See Clinical judgment strategies and operational actions

Atkins v. Virginia (2002), 35-37

Best practices
components, 1, 10
See also Clinical judgment, Professional ethics and standards, Research-based knowledge

Clinical judgment
compared to professional ethics and standards, 1, 6-7
context, 1, 3-5
contraindications, 6
definition, 5-6
framework, 1-2
guidelines, 22-23, 96, 99-101
See also Clinical judgment guidelines incorporating clinical judgment into best practices, 92-96
key points about, 91-92
operational actions, 21-22, 94-97
See also Clinical judgment strategies and operational actions
personal characteristics affecting, 29-30
purpose, 5
relation to best practices, 10
relation to critical thinking, 25-30
relation to professional ethics and professional standards, 6, 8-9
relation to research-based knowledge, 11, 14
situations typically requiring clinical judgment, 15-16, 33
strategies, 17-21, 92-93
See also Clinical judgment strategies and operational actions